5000 Years of Plagues:

A Brief History of Epidemics

James R. Jones, MD, MBA

Revised November 2, 2025

Humans are semi-intelligent mobile platforms designed for the propagation and spread of microorganisms.

Marc Crislip

Author

James R. Jones, MD, MBA, is a physician and healthcare executive with a diverse background that offers a unique blend of expertise in his writing. He graduated from the University of North Texas (BS in Chemistry, 1968), Baylor College of Medicine (MD, 1972), the American Board of Family Practice (Diplomat, 1977), and Southern Methodist University (MBA, 1984). Dr. Jones practiced family medicine for 44 years and was an executive in ten healthcare companies.

Outside of his professional life, he reads, cooks, collects old recipes, and is a seasoned kayaker who has kayaked and canoed over 4,000 miles in rivers, ocean bays, fjords, and swamps.

Books by James R. Jones

Anger
Our Recipes
5000 Years of Plagues
Surviving in Management
A Brief Outline of the History of Medicine
A Contented Life, Practical Advice from Stoicism
Healthcare Contracting for Physician Executives
Camp, Canoe, Kayak – 50 Years of Wilderness Water Trips

amazon.com/author/jamesrjones

Introduction

Plagues and epidemics are not just a part of history — they occur frequently, are deadly, and affect the entire world. We tend to forget them quickly, fail to prepare for the next one, and react with surprise when it occurs.

Malaria devastated the American South until 1952, and in the following decade, 90,000 Americans contracted polio. Influenza recurs every year and will eventually mutate into a more deadly form.

Not only are we vulnerable to 1400 microorganisms that infect humans, but any of the 320,000 viruses that infect animals can also jump species and cause a plague. Increasing numbers of people are crowding the Earth, travel times are decreasing, and epidemics are becoming inevitable.

For example, from 2017 to 2025, twenty-three epidemics occurred, few of which were widely covered in the media.

2017
    Lassa Fever in Nigeria
    Dengue in Pakistan
    Japanese Encephalitis in India
    Dengue in Sri Lanka
2018
    Nipah Virus in India
    The Kivu Ebola Epidemic in the Congo
2019
    Measles in The Congo
    Measles in New Zealand
    Measles in the Philippines
    Measles in Malaysia
    Measles in Samoa
    Dengue in Asia Pacific and Latin America
2019-2022

The COVID-19 Pandemic
2020
    Ebola in the Congo
    Dengue in Singapore
    Yellow Fever in Nigeria
2021
    Mucormycosis (Black Fungus) in India
2022
    Monkeypox Worldwide
    Ebola in Uganda
2023
    Legionella in Poland
    Dengue in Brazil
2023-2025
    World-Wide Mpox
    Sudanese Cholera Epidemic

Table of Contents

8

Infectivity

A disease's reproduction number, R0 ("*R naught*") is the average number of people infected by a single victim. R0 involves complex calculations and careful interpretation.

Diseases ranked by approximate R0:

Measles	15
Chickenpox	11
Mumps	11
Covid-19, Delta	8
Pertussis	6
Polio	6
Rubella	6
Smallpox	5
COVID-19 (original strain)	4
Common Cold	3
Diphtheria	3
Ebola	2
1918 Spanish Flu	2
2009 Influenza	2
Tuberculosis	2
SARS	1
MERS	1

Lethality

The case fatality rate is the percentage of people diagnosed with a disease who die from it. It does not include undiagnosed or asymptomatic cases.

Diseases ranked by approximate Case Fatality Rate:

Ebola	90.00%
HIV/AIDS	90.00%
Influenza A, subtype H5N1	60.00%
Pneumonic Plague	60.00%
Tetanus	50.00%
Tuberculosis (*not latent TB*)	43.00%
Bubonic plague	40.00%
MERS	35.00%
Smallpox, *Variola major*	30.00%
Dengue	26.00%
Hantavirus	20.00%
Polio, Adults	20.00%
Typhoid fever	15.00%
SARS	11.00%
Diphtheria	7.00%
Polio, Children	5.00%
Pertussis (*whooping cough*)	4.00%
COVID-19 (2020 estimate)	3.00%
1918 (Spanish) influenza	3.00%
Measles (*rubeola*)	2.00%
Smallpox *Variola Minor*	1.00%
Malaria	0.30%
Asian influenza (1956–58)	0.10%
Hong Kong influenza (1968–69)	0.10%
Typical seasonal influenza A	0.10%
Varicella (*chickenpox*), adults	0.02%
Varicella (*chickenpox*), children	0.00%

Vaccine Effectiveness

Vaccine effectiveness measures how much a vaccination reduces the disease attack rate.

Vaccines ranked by approximate effectiveness:

Tetanus	99%
Ebola	99%
Rubella (Measles)	97%
Diphtheria	95 %
Hib	95%
COVID-19	95%
Hepatitis B	95%
Polio	90%
Pneumococcal (pneumonia)	90%
Hepatitis A	90%
Mumps	80%
Pertussis (Whooping Cough)	80%
Rotavirus	80%
Chickenpox	80%
Influenza	60%

Available Vaccines

https://www.who.int/teams/immunization-vaccines-and-biologicals/diseases

Cholera
COVID-19 (corona virus)
Dengue
Diphtheria
Hepatitis
Haemophilus influenzae type b (Hib)
Human papillomavirus (HPV)
Influenza
Japanese encephalitis
Malaria
Measles
Meningococcal meningitis
Mumps
Pertussis
Pneumococcal disease
Poliomyelitis
Rabies
Rotavirus
Rubella
Tetanus
Tick-borne encephalitis
Tuberculosis
Typhoid
Varicella
Yellow Fever

Seven Plagues

Smallpox

Frightful, capricious, and cruel — with the power over life and death, the ancients viewed smallpox as punishment from vengeful gods. At least seven cultures had gods associated with smallpox, like the African god Sopona of the Yoruba and the Hindu goddess Shitala.

The earliest documented case of smallpox is found in a 3,000-year-old Egyptian mummy from 1145 BCE. The first written records describing the infection date back to 1500 BCE.

The earliest recorded epidemic occurred during the Peloponnesian War (431–404 BCE). The Spartans emerged victorious after smallpox devastated Athens.

Smallpox contributed to Macedonia's rise and Alexander the Great's victories.

From 165 to 180 CE, the disease affected Italy, killing one-third of the population and speeding up the decline of the Western Roman Empire.

Smallpox invaded India in 400 CE. A contemporary medical text described it:

> *The pustules are red, yellow, and white and are accompanied by burning pain. The skin seems studded with grains of rice.*

Smallpox arrived in Europe in 581 CE, establishing a reservoir and spreading worldwide through European exploration and colonization.

The most explicit pre-modern description of smallpox was by the 9th-century Persian physician Muhammad ibn Zakariya al-Razi (Rhazes). He differentiated it from measles and chickenpox in *Kitab fi al-jadari wa-al-hasbah* (*The Book of Smallpox and Measles*).

The term *"smallpox"* arose in Britain in the 1500s to distinguish it from syphilis, known as the *"great"* pox for its horrible sores.

Cortez invaded Mexico in 1519, and Pizarro conquered Peru in 1532. The conquistadors had horses, better weapons, and superior tactics. However, the virus they unknowingly carried caused far more destruction – in Mexico, smallpox killed a quarter of the population and most of the Aztec army. The Spaniards couldn't walk the streets without stepping over the bodies of smallpox victims.

> *Indians died in heaps. In many places, everyone in a house died, and, as it was impossible to bury such a great number, they pulled down the houses over them so that their homes became their tombs.*
> *Motolina*

The impact of smallpox on the Inca Empire was even more devastating. It spread quickly along the efficient and extensive Inca highway system. Within months, the disease killed the Inca ruler and his successors. Within three years, seventy-five percent of the native population had perished miserably.

Exposed to smallpox for the first time, indigenous populations never stood a chance. Smallpox devastated the Americas, killing eighty percent of the Indigenous inhabitants. For two hundred years, it infected every population in the Western Hemisphere.

In 1633, in Massachusetts, the virus struck Native Americans. It killed Mohawks in 1634, circled Lake Ontario in 1636, and devastated the Iroquois by 1679. During the 1770s, smallpox killed thirty percent of West Coast Native Americans. In 1721, practically the entire population of Boston fled to escape smallpox, only to spread it throughout all the Thirteen Colonies.

The Plains Indians' smallpox epidemic (1780-1782) depopulated the region.

> *Families lay unburied in their tents while the few survivors fled to spread the disease.*
>
> **E. E. Rich**

Three-quarters of the Ojibway and Cree died. Peter Kalm described Indigenous villages overrun with wolves feasting on corpses. Smallpox killed fifty percent of Indigenous Australians in the early years of British colonization. It nearly wiped out the aboriginal people of Easter Island.

Jared Diamond's _Guns, Germs, and Steel_ is an excellent analysis of diseases and the development of primitive civilizations.

Smallpox was a major cause of death throughout the 18th century. One out of every seven children born in Russia died from it. It claimed the lives of 400,000 Europeans each year, including five reigning European monarchs.

Smallpox has two forms: Variola Major, with a 30% mortality rate, and the milder Variola Minor, with a 2% mortality rate. Each type confers immunity to both. In 1549, Chinese physicians began "variolation," where pus from a Variola Minor lesion was scratched into healthy skin to induce immunity to Variola Minor and the more deadly Variola Major. Without variolation, 60% of children caught smallpox, and 20% died. Survivors often lived with severe scars. Edward Jenner believed cowpox provided immunity to smallpox. In 1796, he inoculated patients with cowpox pus. Cowpox caused no illness, was non-contagious, and resulted in no scarring, while offering complete immunity against all forms of smallpox. Despite initial resistance from Western medicine, Catherine the Great vaccinated her court and all Russian serfs. Even with an effective vaccine, smallpox continued to claim lives for the next 181 years.

The Franco-Prussian War sparked a pandemic (1870–1875) that resulted in 500,000 deaths. Between 1868 and 1907, India experienced approximately 4.7 million smallpox-related deaths. Between 1926 and 1930, India reported 979,738 cases, with a mortality rate of 42.3%.

During the 20th century, smallpox killed 400 million people. Even in the 1950s, there were 50 million cases of smallpox each year. As recently as 1967, fifteen million people contracted the disease, and two million died.

In the 1970s, the World Health Organization initiated a smallpox eradication program under the leadership of Australian Frank Fenner. His network of consultants trained countries to set up surveillance and containment systems.

The last epidemic of smallpox occurred in former Yugoslavia in 1972. The last Variola major case was in Bangladesh in 1975, and the final Variola minor case occurred in Merca, Somalia, in 1977. In one of humanity's proudest achievements, the world eradicated smallpox in December 1979.

> *The world and its peoples have won freedom from smallpox, a devastating disease sweeping in epidemics through countries from the earliest times, leaving death, blindness, and disfigurement in its wake.*
>
> *W.H.O.*

Tuberculosis

Tuberculosis has co-evolved with humans over millions of years. The earliest evidence of Mycobacterium tuberculosis dates back 18,000 years to bison bones. Prehistoric human skeletons from 7000 BCE display signs of tuberculosis. X-rays of some Egyptian mummies from 3000 BCE show TB of the spine. The earliest evidence of tuberculosis in South America is found in the Paracas-Caverna culture (750 BCE to 100 CE).

Around 460 BCE, Hippocrates wrote that phthisis (the Greek term for tuberculosis) was the most common disease of his time. The symptoms included coughing up blood and fever — it was always fatal.

In _The Canon of Medicine_, Ibn Sina (Avicenna) identified pulmonary tuberculosis as contagious and noted its association with diabetes. He was the first to suggest that it spread through contact with soil and water. He recommended quarantine to limit its spread. Previously, treatments focused on diet. Pliny the Elder described several in his _Natural History_.

Tuberculosis destroys its victims from within, with a bloody cough, fever, pallor, and relentless wasting. Physicians called it consumption, phthisis; scrofula (tuberculosis of the lymphatic system); tabes mesenterica (tuberculosis of the abdomen); lupus vulgaris (tuberculosis of the skin); Pott's disease (tuberculosis of the spine and joints); and miliary tuberculosis (when the infection invades the circulatory system, causing lung lesions that look like millet seeds). Tuberculosis was identified as a single disease in 1820, and Johann Lukas Schönlein named it "_Tuberculosis_" in 1839.

It is impossible to overstate the importance of TB. It was a widespread disease. In 1815, one in four deaths in England was due to tuberculosis; in 1918, tuberculosis accounted for one out of every six deaths in France. During the 20th century, it claimed the lives of one hundred million people. Even with the best medical care, fifty percent of symptomatic victims died within five years.

Throughout human history, one in every seven deaths has been from tuberculosis. It has killed at least one billion people over the millennia.

In 1946, the discovery of streptomycin enabled the treatment and, in some cases, the cure of tuberculosis. Before the introduction of streptomycin, surgeons either collapsed an infected lung or removed lung tissue to reduce bacterial growth and expose the bacteria to drugs in the bloodstream. In 2009, I treated two patients in their 70s, each of whom had one lung removed twenty years earlier to treat tuberculosis.

Currently, two billion people, one-third of the world's population, have TB, most without clinical symptoms. Eight million people become sick each year, and two million die from this ancient disease. In 2016, India reported over 1.8 million active tuberculosis cases.

Malaria

Mosquitoes trapped in 30-million-year-old amber have the Malaria parasite. Malaria has infected humans for so long that evolution has selected human mutations that confer some protection against Malaria: sickle-cell disease, thalassemia, glucose-6-phosphate dehydrogenase deficiency, ovalocytosis, and elliptocytosis.

Female *Anopheles* mosquitoes, infected with the malaria parasite, inject parasitic sporozoites when they bite a human to get blood. The sporozoites travel to the liver. There, they produce thousands of merozoites that infect red blood cells. Inside the red blood cells, merozoites replicate, eventually bursting the infected cells and releasing the merozoites to invade more red blood cells, thereby repeating the cycle. Some merozoites become gametocytes. When a mosquito bites an infected person, gametocytes enter the mosquito and form ookinetes that become sporozoites and travel to the mosquito's salivary glands, ready to infect a new host.

Malaria victims experience repeated cycles of chills, shivering, fever, and sweating. Attacks occur every two days with P. vivax and P. ovale infections, and every three days with P. malariae. The fever caused by P. falciparum generally occurs every 36 hours but can sometimes be continuous.

The Chinese medical text *Huangdi Neijing* describes recurrent fevers associated with enlarged spleens and epidemics. The Sanskrit medical treatise *Sushruta Samhita* (6th Century BCE) describes the symptoms of Malaria. The ancient Greek physicians recognized Malaria. Hippocrates associated intermittent fevers with climatic and environmental conditions and classified them according to their periodicity. Leonardo Bruni first used the term '*mal' aria*' (bad air) in 1476. European settlers and enslaved

African Captives brought Anopheles mosquitoes and Malaria to the Americas in the 16th Century.

Agostino Salumbrino observed Quechua Indians using the quinine-containing bark of the cinchona tree for malaria-induced shivering. It was introduced into European medicine by Barnabé de Cobo. He was in Spain in 1582; he died in Lima, Peru, in 1657. De Cobo was a Spanish Jesuit missionary and writer who wrote a description of cinchona bark and brought some to Europe in 1632. In 1820, Pelletier and Caventou isolated cinchonine and quinine from the bark, enabling the production of standardized doses of the active ingredients.

Charles Ledger smuggled cinchona seeds out of Bolivia (their export was illegal) and sold them to the Dutch. In 1865, the Dutch government planted 20,000 Cinchona ledgeriana trees in Java. By the end of the Nineteenth Century, the Dutch had a worldwide monopoly of quinine in one of the first "*Big Pharma*" operations.

In 1850, William Henry Perkin tried to synthesize quinine. He accidentally produced mauve, a synthetic dye excellent for staining tissues and blood. This unintended result was the key to finding and studying the malaria parasite. Using the dye to stain slides, Alphonse Laveran, a French military surgeon, found the parasites in victims' red blood cells using the stain. He received the Nobel prize in 1907.

Golgi found that the parasites reproduced and multiplied simultaneously at regular intervals. These divisions caused the attacks of fever.

In Secunderabad, India, Sir Ronald Ross proved in 1897 that mosquitoes transmit Malaria. Ross, a British officer in the Indian Medical Service, was the first to demonstrate that malaria parasites are transmitted by mosquitoes. Furthermore, Ross proved that mosquitoes transmitted malaria parasites from bird to bird. He solved the mystery of malaria transmission. Ross received the Nobel prize in 1902.

Grassi showed that only Anopheles mosquitoes could transmit human Malaria.

Because patients with syphilis improved when they suffered a high fever, Julius Wagner-Jauregg tried infecting neurosyphilis patients with P. vivax Malaria. Four bouts of fever killed the temperature-sensitive Treponema pallidum and stopped the progression of neurosyphilis. Then, quinine cured the Malaria infection. Julius Wagner-Jauregg received the 1927 Nobel Prize for using Malaria to treat dementia paralytica.

Müller discovered the insecticidal properties of DDT in 1939, earning the Nobel Prize in 1948. In 1947, the National Malaria Eradication Program implemented the widespread use of DDT for mosquito control, ultimately eradicating malaria from the U.S.

In the 1960s, Rachel Clark's book *Silent Spring* pointed out that DDT was causing brittle eggshells in songbirds in the U.S. and had caused a steep drop in the songbird population. A public outcry led to a ban on DDT use worldwide, and the Endangered Species Act, which saved the bald eagle and the peregrine falcon from extinction.

DDT, the most effective anti-mosquito agent known, was phased out of use. The unintended result was a significant rise in malaria deaths in less developed countries. In 2016, DDT was reintroduced in the fight against malaria.

Malaria continues to infect impoverished areas with poor drainage, where Anopheles mosquitoes easily breed. Houses without air conditioning or screens cannot keep mosquitoes out. If people cannot afford DDT, bug repellents, or nets, mosquitoes are free to come and go as they please.

One million people die from malaria each year, most of whom are under five years old, and ninety percent of these deaths occur in Sub-Saharan Africa. Forty percent of the world's population lives in regions affected by malaria. In 2016, malaria infected 250 million new people.

Drugs become less effective against malaria as the parasite evolves. On January 22, 2024, Cameroon started administering RTS,S/AS01, the first malaria vaccine used in a national immunization program. On December 21, 2023, the WHO prequalified a second malaria vaccine, R21/Matrix-M.

Rabies

The Mesopotamian Codex of Eshnunna mentions Rabies in 1930 BCE. If a person bitten by a rabid dog died, the dog's owner paid a fine.

Roman, Scribonius Largus, treated rabies with hyena skin. Antaeus recommended a hanged man's skull.

The disease originated in the Old World, spread to Boston in 1768, and then across North America.

Rabies was prevalent in 19th-century France and Belgium. People bitten by a rabid dog often committed suicide before local villagers killed them. So, it was easy for Louis Pasteur to find volunteers for his experiments.

Louis Pasteur and Émile Roux created the rabies vaccine in 1885. On 6 July 1885, nine-year-old Joseph Meister (1876–1940) endured thirteen injections over ten days and became the first human to survive a rabid dog's bite.

As of 2021, rabies still kills at least 60,000 people in Africa and Asia each year. Most cases of dog bites occur in impoverished areas. Half of the victims are children.

The Black Death

The worldwide Black Death was the deadliest plague in history, killing at least seventy-five million people from 1331 to 1353 CE.

From Asia, it traveled the Silk Road to Crimea. Fleas living on ship rats carried it throughout the Mediterranean to Africa, Western Asia, and Europe. It killed 30 million — sixty percent of the population.

Bubonic Plague is spread by fleabites and manifests in skin lesions (bubos). Pneumonic Plague spreads by respiratory droplets, attacks the lungs, and kills its victims swiftly.

Father abandoned child, wife, husband, one brother, another; for this illness seemed to strike through the breath and sight. And so, they died. And none could be found to bury the dead for money or friendship. Members of a household brought their dead to a ditch as best they could, without a priest, without divine offices ... great pits were dug and piled deep with the multitude of dead. And they died by the hundreds both day and night ... And as soon as those ditches were filled, more were dug ... And I, Agnolo di Tura ... buried my five children with my own hands. And no one who wept for any death, for all awaited death. And so many died that all believed it was the end of the world.
Agnolo di Tura, May 1348, Siena,

Bubonic and Pneumonic Plague still kill. There are 1,000 to 3,000 cases every year. In 2014, Madagascar suffered 119 instances, with forty deaths.

The Spanish Flu

From March 1918 to June 1920, the Spanish Flu spread to every part of the world, even the Arctic and remote Pacific islands. The first wave, in early March, resembled the typical flu. However, by August, the virus had mutated into a much deadlier form, and its victims were healthy young adults.

Without vaccines or antibiotics, the only "treatments" were isolation, quarantine, hand washing, disinfectants, and bans on public gatherings. However, governments suppressed reports of the flu to maintain post-war morale. Returning soldiers with the flu were sent to overcrowded hospitals, which further spread the disease.

This holocaust may have killed more people than the Black Death. One-third of the world's population was infected. At least fifty million people died worldwide, most within six months. Seventeen million died in India, five percent of the total population. In Japan, 390,000 perished. In the U.S., the flu claimed 500,000 lives. In Britain, the death toll was 250,000. In France, 400,000 died. Entire native villages in Alaska vanished completely.

Symptoms were unusual, and the Spanish flu was often misdiagnosed as dengue, cholera, or typhoid. Complications included bleeding from the nose, stomach, intestines, and ears. Death resulted from severe hemorrhaging and lung edema.

In 1933, the influenza A virus was isolated. A vaccine became available in 1944, and by 1950, vaccination had become routine.

In 1998, Johan Hultin recovered DNA samples from a Native Alaskan woman's frozen corpse buried in permafrost for eighty years. Finally, researchers could analyze the genetic structure of the 1918 virus. In 2000, Sir John Skehel and Professor Ian Wilson synthesized the hemagglutinin protein, which is responsible for its lethality. In 2005, researchers at the Mount Sinai School of Medicine in New York completely reconstructed the genetic sequence of the 1918 influenza. It was a subtype of avian H1N1. The H1N1 influenza A virus also caused the 2009 swine flu pandemic.

Coronaviruses

Virologists isolated Coronaviruses from animals in the 1960s. They cause colds, pneumonia, diarrhea, and bronchitis in chickens, pigs, cows, cats, dogs, civets, ferrets, mice, camels, and bats. As of 2021, Coronaviruses have jumped from animals to humans three times.

SARS

From 2002 to 2004, SARS-CoV caused an epidemic of *Severe Acute Respiratory Syndrome*. Over 8,000 people were infected, and 10 percent died.

MERS

In 2012, the Coronavirus MERS-CoV caused *Middle East Respiratory Syndrome*. By 2019, 2468 cases of **MERS** had killed 851, a mortality rate of 35%. Sporadic cases still occur.

COVID-19

In 2015, Vineet D. Menachery, Boyd L. Yount Jr., et al. published an article in Nature Medicine (volume 21, number 12, December 2015), warning that coronavirus viruses can replicate in humans and that there was a high potential risk of a future SARS or MERS epidemic. Despite the warning, no country began preparing for the possibility of such an epidemic.

In September 2019, 959 Italian patients had blood samples collected and stored for future research. In March 2021, Giovanni Apolone, Emanuele Montomoli, and Alessandro Manenti examined the samples and detected SARS-CoV-2 (COVID-19) antibodies in 111 samples.

Unexpected detection of SARS-CoV-2 antibodies in pre-pandemic Italy https://journals.sagepub.com/doi/full/10. 1177/0300891620974755 Tumori. 2021 Mar 22:300891620987756. https://doi.org/10.1177/03008916209747 55

Thus, *in retrospect*, SARS-CoV-2 <u>may</u> have already been in Italy three months *before* the world's first case was identified.

The world first learned about COVID-19 on December 8, 2019. That day, in Wuhan, China, a woman developed an unusual pneumonia and spread it to others. On December 26, 2019, Jixian Zhang, MD, director of the Respiratory and Critical Care department at Hubei Provincial Hospital, treated four cases of the new pneumonia, all from the same family. She reported the situation to the local CDC. Three more patients appeared on December 30, 2019, and China's CDC notified WHO on December 31, 2019. By January 7, 2020, scientists in China had fully sequenced the RNA of the mutated coronavirus, known as SARS-CoV-2.

Despite unprecedented quarantine measures in China and other countries, the disease quickly spread worldwide. A traveler from Wuhan was the first U.S. case in January 2020.

In December 2019, the mutated Coronavirus SARS-CoV-2 triggered the COVID-19 pandemic. It spread from China globally, killing millions and paralyzing the world economy.

In March, 163 countries reported 250,000 cases with 10,000 deaths. By May, it had infected six million people, with 360,000 deaths. There were 59 million cases and 1.4 million deaths worldwide by November.

The World Health Organization estimated a need for two billion doses of a COVID-19 vaccine. In the U.S., Operation Warp Speed funded $10 billion for 300 million vaccine doses. By December 2020, forty-four vaccines were being tested for initial safety and dosage, nineteen were in expanded safety trials, eighteen were conducting large-scale efficacy tests, and five were in limited use. The U.S. approved two vaccines in December and began widespread vaccinations in January 2021.

The COVID-19 vaccines are among the most important achievements in medical history due to their speed, technological progress, and global influence. The effort involved unmatched international cooperation between governments, private companies, and scientists. The first effective vaccines by Pfizer-BioNTech and Moderna were developed, tested, approved, and distributed in less than a year — a feat never before achieved for a new virus. The mRNA vaccine platforms were revolutionary, opening new possibilities for future vaccines against cancer, flu, and RSV. Over 13 billion doses have been administered worldwide — the largest vaccination campaign in human history. Reliable studies estimate that the vaccines saved 15–20 million lives in 2021 alone and prevented healthcare system failures in many countries.

As of June 2021, eighteen months into the pandemic, 34 million documented USA cases had resulted in 600,000 deaths. Worldwide, at least 200 million cases caused 4 million deaths. A massive effort vaccinated forty percent (135 million) of the U.S. population, and daily deaths dropped to *"only"* 700. However, 94% of the world remained unvaccinated.

The massive global reservoir of COVID-19 infections produced countless mutations. For example, Delta emerged in India in December 2020 and quickly spread through that country and Great Britain before reaching the U.S., where it rapidly surged.

Delta soon accounted for over 99% of COVID-19 cases, resulting in a sharp rise in hospitalizations. Additionally, Delta was much more contagious than the original strain, with an R0 of nearly eight.

By January 2021, COVID-19 had infected 100 million people worldwide, resulting in two million deaths. The United States had 23 million infections and 380,000 deaths.

As of July 11, 2022, COVID-19 has caused over 6 million deaths.

Scientists rushed forty-four vaccines into testing, and widespread vaccinations began in early 2021.

There was no effective treatment or cure available during the early years of the pandemic. In 2021, the European Medicines Agency's Committee for Medicinal Products for Human Use approved Paxlovid (nirmatrelvir plus ritonavir) for the treatment of adults. Later, the FDA in the US granted it Emergency Use Authorization.

Opportunists spread false information about the disease and vaccines across social media.

After December 2020, COVID-19 vaccines were widely distributed. According to a June 2022 study, COVID-19 vaccines likely prevented 17 million deaths between 2020 and 2021.

As of November 2022, COVID-19 had caused 16 million excess deaths.

The COVID-19 pandemic caused global social and economic disruption, leading to the most significant recession since the Great Depression. Additionally, there were widespread shortages of supplies and food.

More to Come

Four coronavirus variants — 229E, OC43, NL63, and HKU1 — can infect humans but have not caused epidemics — yet. However, they inevitably will.

7000 BCE to 3000 BCE

The world's population was five million, and life expectancy at birth was under twenty years.

3400 BCE – Tuberculosis and the Pharaohs

The mummy of Nesperehan displays spinal tuberculosis with a collapsed vertebra, causing kyphosis. A large tuberculosis abscess of the psoas muscle is also present.

3000 BCE to 1000 BCE

The world's population increased from fourteen million to twenty-seven million. Life expectancy at birth was twenty-five years.

1500 BCE – Smallpox in India

Ancient medical writings from India have the earliest known descriptions of smallpox.

1145 BCE – Smallpox and Ramses the Fifth

Lesions on the face of the mummy of Ramses the Fifth indicate that he died from smallpox. He is one of the earliest known victims of the disease.

1122 BCE – Smallpox in China

Chinese medical texts describe a condition that likely was smallpox.

1000 BCE to 1000 CE

The world population grew from fifty million to 275 million. Life expectancy at birth increased to twenty-eight years. The historical record of epidemics during this period is sparse.

430 BCE – The Plague of Athens

During the Peloponnesian War, plagues decimated Athens in 430, 429, and 427 BCE. Recurrences continued until 404 BCE, resulting in the deaths of two-thirds of the population. Thousands of soldiers and sailors died, along with the great Athenian general, Pericles. The smoke from funeral pyres frightened the Spartans so much that they stopped their attacks and withdrew. Thucydides, who caught the plague but survived, wrote that Athens did not fully recover for fifteen years. Modern experts believe the disease was smallpox or a hemorrhagic fever similar to today's Ebola.

The ears besieged with buzzings, the respiration rapid or ponderous, the neck bedewed with glistening beads of sweat, the saliva thin and scanty, salty and flecked with yellow. Ghastly ulcers and black discharge from the bowels or else a flux of purulent blood. Their languid limbs half dead, caked with filth, covered with rags.
Lucretius, quoting Thucydides.
De rerum natura (69 BCE)

165–180 CE – Antonine Plague

The Antonine Plague, also known as the Plague of Galen, who described it, arrived in the Roman Empire with troops returning from the Middle East. It was either smallpox or measles. The plague first appeared during the Roman siege of Seleucia in 165. Thousands died across the empire. It struck again in 189 CE, killing 2,000 people daily in Rome. Total deaths reached five million, and in some regions, one-third of the population was wiped out.

The Antonine Plague struck Rome repeatedly from 165 to 180 CE. In 174 CE, it killed 2,000 a day in Rome and devastated the Roman army. The Greek physician, philosopher, and writer Galen described it as having a long duration, accompanied by fever, diarrhea, pharyngitis, and a skin rash suggestive of smallpox.

249 CE – Plague of Cyprian

The Plague of Cyprian ravaged the Roman Empire from 249 to 262 CE. Plausible causes include smallpox, influenza, and hemorrhagic fever.

340 CE – Measles versus Smallpox

Chinese alchemist Ko Hung described the differences between smallpox and measles.

400 CE – Smallpox in India

Smallpox invaded India in 400 CE. A text for the time describes the disease:

The pustules are red, yellow, and white, and they are accompanied by burning pain. The skin seems studded with grains of rice.

541 CE – The Plague of Justinian

The Plague of Justinian afflicted the Eastern Roman Empire, Constantinople, and cities around the Mediterranean. It recurred repeatedly for two hundred years and killed twenty-five million people. Finally, in 2013, researchers confirmed the cause as Yersinia pestis, Bubonic, and Pneumonic Plague — the Black Death.

590 CE – The Roman Plague

Another plague struck the city of Rome. It was probably smallpox

664 CE – The Yellow Plague of Britain

This plague disrupted the British Isles for twenty-five years, resulting in widespread mortality. Its cause is still unknown.

735–737 CE – Smallpox in Japan

The epidemic killed one-third of Japan's population.

1000 CE to 1500 CE

The world's population increased to 450 million. Life expectancy at birth reached thirty years.

1347–1353 – The Black Death

Pasteurella Pestis spread from Central Asia into Europe, killing sixty percent of the European population (estimated at 50 million) in just six years. Worldwide deaths were probably around seventy-five million. The Black Death reduced the world population to four hundred million.

Fleabites spread the Bubonic Plague, which starts with skin lesions (bubos). Pneumonic Plague spreads by respiratory droplets and attacks the lungs. It is swiftly fatal.

> *There came into the noble city of Florence a deadly pestilence where it destroyed countless lives. That horrible plague began with swellings in the groin and armpit, some of which were as big as apples and some of which were shaped like eggs, some were small, and others were large. The fatal bubos (swellings) would begin to spread, and within a short while, the body would be covered with dark and livid spots; these were certain indications of coming death.*
> **Boccaccio – The Decameron**

Europe was devastated; fields lay untended, and flocks and herds wandered loose. Religious fanatics scourged themselves for their sins. Anonymous "plague tracts" recommended bloodletting, drinking vinegar, and fleeing as far as possible — which only spread the disease wider.

Bubonic and Pneumonic Plague still kill. In 2014, Madagascar suffered 119 cases, with forty deaths.

1476 – Malaria Named

Leonardo Bruni used the Italian term *"bad air"* (mal'aria) to describe the disease. Read the section on Malaria.

1492 to 1600 – The Columbian Exchange

Beginning with Columbus's voyages of discovery, a widespread exchange of plants, animals, precious metals, goods, culture, human populations, technology, ideas, and diseases occurred between the Americas and the Old World.

Before 1492, Indigenous peoples in the Americas numbered 54 million. Ninety percent (48 million) were killed in the next 100 years by European and African diseases such as smallpox, measles, typhoid fever, bubonic plague, cholera, yellow fever, malaria, diphtheria, and influenza.

1494 – Syphilis in Europe

Syphilis was unknown until the voyages of Christopher Columbus. Modern researchers believe sailors caught bejel and yaws in Guyana and carried the spirochetes back to Europe, where they combined and mutated into the scourge of syphilis.

In 1495, Charles VIII of France laid siege to Naples, and this new, terrible plague struck. First, it infected the soldiers besieging the city. Then, soldiers returning home spread it to every bed in Europe.

Pustules (poxes) covered sufferers from their heads to their toes. Dying flesh fell off faces, and death followed within months. In 1505, the disease decimated China. By 1546, it evolved into a milder illness with the symptoms known today.

Now, syphilis is preventable and curable, but in 2018, there were 115,000 cases in the US and 1300 in newborn babies.

1500 to 1750

The world's population was six hundred million. Life expectancy at birth was thirty-three years.

1500 – Smallpox Named

The term <u>small</u>pox came into use in Britain in the 1500s to distinguish it from syphilis, which was called the "<u>great</u>" pox because of the gigantic size of its horrible skin ulcers.

1519 – Smallpox in Mexico

In 1519, Cortez landed in Mexico, and smallpox landed with them. It destroyed the Aztec army and a quarter of the population. The Spaniards could not walk the streets without stepping on the bodies of smallpox victims.

> *Indians died in heaps. In many places, everyone in a house died, and, as it was impossible to bury such a great number, they pulled down the houses over them so that their homes became their tombs.*
> *Motolina*

1525 – Smallpox in India

An epidemic swept India.

1532 – Smallpox in Peru

Pizzaro invaded Peru in 1532. Within months, the disease killed the Inca ruler and his successors. Within three years, seventy-five percent of the native population had died.

1576–1580 – Cocoliztli Epidemic in Mexico

Millions died from high fevers and bleeding in the worst epidemic in Mexico's history. Genomic studies identify *Salmonella Paratyphi C* as the cause.

1578 – Whooping Cough in Paris

Guillaume de Baillou studied the epidemics tormenting Paris, producing the first clinical description of pertussis (whooping cough).

1592 – Plague in London

During London's last major outbreak of Bubonic and Pneumonic Plague, the Black Death claimed 15,000 lives in the City of London and 4,900 in the surrounding areas.

1612 – Typhoid Fever Kills the Prince

Henry, Prince of Wales, the oldest son of King James I, died at age eighteen from typhoid fever. It is the earliest documented case in English history.

1613 – Diphtheria in Spain

Spaniards called this epidemic "*El Año de los Garotillos*" ("*the year of the strangulations*").

1616 – Unknown Epidemic in New England

This mysterious disease killed thirty percent of settlers and the local Wampanoag natives.

1625 – Smallpox in Canada

French Jesuits in Canada wrote:

> *Since we arrived in these lands, those natives who had been the nearest to us have been the most ruined by smallpox, and whole villages of those who had received us are now utterly exterminated.*

1629 – Black Death in Milan

Bubonic and Pneumonic Plague killed twenty-five percent of the population in Italy. One million died.

1633 – Smallpox in Massachusetts

Settlers and Native Americans died, including twenty of the original colonists from the Mayflower and the only physician.

1634 – Smallpox among the Mohawks

1636 – Smallpox around Lake Ontario

1647–1652 – Black Death in Seville

Bubonic and Pneumonic Plague killed twenty-five percent of Seville's population.

1657 – Measles in Boston

1659 – Diphtheria in Boston

1661 – Smallpox, China, and Variolation

Chinese Emperor Fu-lin died of smallpox, but his son survived and later became Emperor K'ang, supporting variolation against smallpox.

> *It has saved the lives and health of millions of men. This is an extremely important thing, of which I am very proud.*

1665 – Black Death in London

The Great Plague of London killed a quarter of the city's population. The resurgence of the Bubonic and Pneumonic

Plagues began in China in 1331, spread globally, and continued to kill victims until 1750.

1679 – Smallpox among the Iroquois

Count de Frontenac Louis de Buade noted:

> *The Indian Plague desolates them to such a degree that they think no longer of war but only of mourning the dead, of whom there is an immense number.*

1694 – Smallpox and the Queen

Queen Mary II of England, age 32, died of smallpox in 1694.

1699 – Yellow Fever in America

Outbreaks of Yellow Fever swept through the colonies.

1707 – Smallpox in Iceland

Smallpox killed 18,000 in Iceland, one-third of the population.

1710 – Black Death in Sweden

The Great Northern War (1700–1721) led to outbreaks of bubonic and pneumonic plague in the Baltic region and Europe. They killed two-thirds of the population, leaving farms and villages abandoned. It was another outbreak of the pandemic that began in Central Asia.

1713 – Measles in Boston.

Measles killed Cotton Mather's wife, his newborn twins, a daughter, and the family servant in two short weeks.

1721 – Smallpox in Boston

Boston's Smallpox epidemic killed 844. However, of 248 Bostonians variolated by Doctor Zabdiel Boylston, 242 lived. The population of Boston fled the city, spreading the virus to the rest of the Thirteen Colonies.

Doctor Boylston was the first physician to perform smallpox variolations in North America. He was the first American doctor to remove gallbladder stones (1710) and a breast tumor (1718).

1732 – Scrapie in Sheep

In the 18th century, sheep imported from Spain were observed to have and transmit a disease called scrapie to other sheep and goats. Affected animals would "*lie down, bite at their feet and legs, rub their backs against posts, fail to thrive, stop feeding, and finally become lame.*" Scrapie is an invariably fatal, degenerative neurological disease of sheep and goats. It is one of several transmissible spongiform encephalopathies (TSEs) and is believed to be caused by a prion.

Scrapie does not seem to be transmissible to humans. However, it has been experimentally transmitted to humanized transgenic mice and non-human primates in laboratory settings.

1738 – Black Death in the Balkans

An outbreak of the Bubonic and Pneumonic Plague killed fifty thousand.

1735 – Diphtheria in New England

Entire families perished, and many lost three out of four children. One town in New Hampshire lost every third child under the age of ten.

1740 – Rubella: The German Measles

German physician Friedrich Hoffmann described rubella.

1750 to 1800

The world's population was nine hundred million. Life expectancy at birth was thirty-five years.

1768 – Smallpox and the Czarina

Physician Thomas Dimsdale inoculated Catherine the Great of Russia against Smallpox in 1768. He used the variolation method. Relays of horses stood by in case Catherine died and Dimsdale had to escape. The results were a success. Catherine suffered a mild illness and recovered. Dimsdale received £10,000, a pension, and a Barony.

1770 – Black Death in Russia

An outbreak of the Bubonic and Pneumonic Plague killed 100,000 Russians, half of them in Moscow.

1777 – Smallpox and George Washington

George Washington ordered mandatory variolation for troops unless they had previously survived smallpox.

1780 – Smallpox on The Great Plains

The Plains Indians' smallpox epidemic decimated the native population from 1780 to 1782.

1767 – Smallpox or Chickenpox?

English physician William Heberden distinguished chickenpox from smallpox and noted that those who had previously had chickenpox could not have it again.

1775–1782 – Smallpox in America

Smallpox infected both sides during the siege of Boston, and enslaved escapees spread it to Texas, New Orleans, and Mexico. The deadly disease spread across the Great Plains to the Pacific Coast and even reached Alaska.

From the Pueblos of New Mexico to trading posts on Hudson's Bay, smallpox destroyed every indigenous tribe in North America.

Variolation vs. Smallpox

There are two forms of smallpox: Variola Minor has a two percent mortality rate. Variola Major kills thirty percent of those infected. Each provides immunity against both types if the patient survives.

In naturally acquired smallpox, inhaled viral particles infect numerous sites in the lungs simultaneously. As a result, the virus multiplies quickly at multiple locations, producing vast amounts of virus particles that overwhelm the body's immune response before it can produce antibodies.

In Variolation, a tiny amount of pus from a skin lesion on a patient with Variola Minor is *"pricked"* (inoculated) into the recipient's skin. As a result, the infection spreads slowly from only one spot, allowing the patients' rising immunity to stop the disease and prevent death.

Smallpox caused by variolation is milder than the epidemic form and has a much lower death rate. An inoculated person is immune to both types of smallpox.

The earliest recorded instance of smallpox variolation occurred in China in 1549, as documented in Wan Quan's _Douzhen Xinfa_. Yu Chang also described it in his _book Notes on My Judgment_, published in 1643.

A Case of childhood smallpox permanently scarred the remarkable Lady Mary Wortley Montagu. She was very interested in using it to protect her children after witnessing variolation succeed in Constantinople in 1718. She asked the embassy surgeon, Charles Maitland, to use it on her son. Maitland tested Variolation on six English prisoners condemned to death, who agreed to be test subjects in exchange for their freedom. Everyone survived. The practice spread across European royal families, but it was adopted by the public only gradually.

In Boston in 1721, Zabdiel Boylston variolated two enslaved servants and his son. Later, he inoculated 300 people during a smallpox epidemic in Boston, with only six fatalities. Sadly, the death rate among unvaccinated Bostonians was twenty percent.

The drawbacks of variolation were that every vaccinated child became sick, was contagious while ill, and a few died. However, sixty percent of children contracted smallpox without variolation, twenty percent of the infected died, and all the survivors were left with disfiguring scars.

1793 – Yellow Fever in Philadelphia

Yellow fever infected 11,000 people in Philadelphia, and 1,000 died. Benjamin Rush's (1745-1813) account of the epidemic describes absolute horror.

1797 – Vaccination vs. Smallpox

Edward Jenner hypothesized that cowpox gave immunity to smallpox. In 1796, he took fluid from Cowpox pustules on milkmaid Sarah Nelmes' hand and injected it into James Phelps. As a result, Phelps became immune to Variola Minor. Jenner then inoculated his children with cowpox and showed that they became immune to smallpox.

Jenner's method was better than variolation. Inoculated patients did not get sick or spread illness and only had scars at the injection site. English medicine rejected Jenner's approach. However, Catherine the Great hired him to vaccinate her entire Royal Court and stop smallpox from killing Russian serfs.

Humanity eradicated smallpox from our planet one hundred eighty-one years after Jenner's vaccine discovery.

1800 to 1850

The world's population was 1.2 billion.

1817–1824 – First Cholera Pandemic

The first Asiatic cholera pandemic began near Calcutta. It spread throughout South and Southeast Asia to the Middle East, Africa, and the Mediterranean. Hundreds of thousands died. It would not be until later epidemics of Cholera that it would ravage Europe and the Americas.

When the epidemic reached Russia, they implemented an anti-cholera program that inspired similar European efforts. As a result, the disease transmission stopped after a cold winter killed the bacteria in water supplies.

1826 – Malaria in Holland

A malaria epidemic killed 2,844 people, ten percent of the population of Groningen.

1826–1837 – Second Cholera Pandemic

Cholera spread from India into Asia, Europe, Great Britain, the Americas, China, and Japan. Hundreds of thousands died.

1836–1840 – Smallpox on the Great Plains

Epidemics spread along the Missouri River and killed more than 17,000 Indigenous people; entire tribes became extinct. Only twenty-seven Mandans survived.

1846–1860 – Third Cholera Pandemic

The third outbreak of Cholera from India reached far beyond its borders. In Russia, one million people died. The epidemic in London killed 10,000.

1847 – Typhus in Canada

Twenty thousand people died in Montreal, Kingston, Grosse Isle, Toronto, and Saint John.

1850 to 1900

The world's population was 1.6 billion. Life expectancy at birth was forty years.

1853 – Smallpox and the United Kingdom Vaccination Act

The act made smallpox vaccination mandatory in the first three months of an infant's life.

1854 – John Snow and the Pump Handle

In August 1854, London experienced an epidemic of Cholera. John Snow mapped residents who died from Cholera and found they drew their water from a public well on Broad Street. He removed the pump's handle on September 8, 1854, and the epidemic stopped. Snow later discovered that the well was only three feet from an old cesspit, leaking fecal bacteria, adding weight to his theory that cholera was a waterborne contagious disease.

Snow's studies and his removal of the pump handle became a model for modern epidemiology. Every year, during the *Annual Pump Handle Lecture* in England, members of the John Snow Society ceremonially remove and then replace a pump handle.

1855 – Black Death in China

The Third Bubonic and Pneumonic Plague Pandemic started in China in 1855 and spread worldwide. Twelve million people died in India and China, with ten million in India alone. This pandemic remained active until 1960.

1863 – Smallpox and President Lincoln

Hours after delivering the Gettysburg Address, President Lincoln contracted smallpox in 1863. According to his valet, he experienced fatigue, fever, and a rash. His doctor, Dr.. Robert K.. Stone, confirmed it was varioloid — a milder form of smallpox seen in people who had been previously exposed or vaccinated. Lincoln was confined to bed for about three weeks. His condition was never life-threatening, although he was isolated to prevent infecting others. His valet, William H.. Johnson, who helped care for him, caught smallpox and died from it. Lincoln recovered completely and resumed his presidential duties by December 1863.

For once in my life as President, I find myself in a position to give everybody something.

1863–1875 – Fourth Cholera Pandemic

The fourth cholera pandemic spread from India to Mecca, killing 30,000. Cholera then hit the Middle East, Russia, Europe, Africa, and North America. Travelers spread it to port cities and inland waterways. It reached Africa in 1865, killing 70,000 in Zanzibar and then 90,000 in Russia. During the Austro-Prussian War (1866), Cholera killed 165,000. In 1867, Italy lost 113,000, and 80,000 died in Algeria. Outbreaks killed 50,000 as Cholera spread along the Mississippi River.

1870 – Smallpox and the Franco–Prussian War

The Franco-Prussian War triggered a smallpox pandemic (1870–1875) that claimed 500,000 lives.

1875 – The Ship HMS Dido Lands in Fiji

A third of the island's population, 20,000 people, died in the following measles epidemic.

1878 – Yellow Fever in the Mississippi Valley

Thirteen thousand people died.

1881 – Mosquitos Carry Yellow Fever

Juan Carlos Finlay y de Barrés (1833–1915) presented a paper to Havana's Academy of Sciences: *The Mosquito Hypothetically Considered as the Transmitting Agent of Yellow Fever*.

1881–1896 – Fifth Cholera Epidemic

The world's fifth cholera pandemic spread to Asia, Africa, France, Germany, Russia, and South America.

1882 – Anti-Vaccination League of America

At their first annual meeting in New York, the league reaffirmed its belief that filth causes smallpox.

1884 – Vaccine vs. Cholera.

Scientists developed the first vaccines against Cholera in the 1800s. In the 1990s, researchers produced an oral cholera vaccine.

1885 – Intubation for Diphtheria

American physician Joseph P. O'Dwyer (1841–1898) refined intubation to open the larynx in Diphtheria patients.

1885 – Rabies Vaccine

Louis Pasteur and Émile Roux created a rabies vaccine, and on July 6, 1885, nine-year-old Joseph Meister (1876–1940) received it. He was the first human in history to survive the bite of a rabid dog.

1889 – Asiatic Flu Pandemic

The 1889–1890 flu pandemic killed one million people worldwide. It was probably the Influenza A virus subtype H3N8.

1890 – Vaccine vs. Tetanus

German scientists led by Emil von Behring created a Tetanus vaccine in 1890.

1894 – Diphtheria Antitoxin in America

Cincinnati physicians G. J. Hermann, MD, and Charles Waugh Reynolds, MD, saved a child with Diphtheria by injecting Diphtheria antitoxin.

1896 – Vaccine vs. Typhoid Fever

Richard Pfeiffer and Wilhelm Kolle demonstrated that inoculation with killed typhoid bacteria provides immunity against typhoid fever.

The United States licenses two Typhoid vaccines. Ty21a is a live, attenuated oral vaccine that provides protection for three years; the injected Vi capsular polysaccharide vaccine offers protection for several years. The typhoid-conjugate vaccine protects for five years but is not available in the United States.

Twenty-one million cases of typhoid fever, with 220,000 deaths, still occur worldwide every year.

1897 – Vaccine vs. The Black Death

Scientists made a vaccine from killed bacteria in 1890. Current bubonic plague vaccines use live attenuated bacilli or recombination proteins.

1898 – Viruses Discovered

The Dutch microbiologist Martinus Beijerinck filtered solutions through a porcelain water filter until no bacteria were present. Instead, he found a previously unknown infectious agent that could only reproduce inside cells. He named it a *virus*.

Friedrich Loeffler and Paul Frosch proved that the virus causing foot-and-mouth disease could pass through a bacteria-proof filter.

By 2021, researchers had characterized more than 2,000 viruses. Current estimates indicate that there are approximately 300,000 mammalian viruses, of which at least 200 cause human disease.

1899–1923 – Sixth Cholera Pandemic

The world's sixth cholera pandemic followed the usual pattern. It began in India, where 800,000 died, spreading to the Middle East, Africa, Eastern Europe, and Russia.

1900 to 1925

The world's population was two billion.

1900 – Simian Immunodeficiency Virus

Researchers believe that, in the 1900s, the simian immunodeficiency virus infected humans in central Africa and later spread worldwide to become the HIV pandemic.

1901 – No Mosquitos, No Yellow Fever

In 1901, Walter Reed (1851–1902) published evidence that mosquitoes transmit yellow fever. Carlos J. Finley of Havana, Cuba, had previously proposed this vector. Reed conducted well-conceived experiments on human subjects that conclusively proved the theory.

In 1901, William C. Gorgas eradicated yellow fever in Havana in just ninety days. In 1903, Juan Guiteras freed Laredo, Texas, of the disease. In 1914, Dr. Gorgas reduced Yellow Fever in Panama to a minor nuisance, allowing the completion of the Canal. By 1928, a vaccine was available.

1901 – Antiserum Nobel Prize

The 1901 Nobel Prize went to Emil Adolf von Behring for Diphtheria antiserum therapy, finally giving physicians a weapon against the illness.

1902 – Nobel Prize for Malaria Research

The 1902 Nobel Prize in Medicine was awarded to the eccentric and polymathic scientist Ronald Ross for discovering the complete life cycle of the malaria parasite.

Ross raised mosquitoes from larvae and infected them with the parasite. Then, he demonstrated that the mosquito salivary gland stores parasites and releases them during biting. Finally, he confirmed that mosquitoes transmit malaria parasites from infected birds to healthy ones.

Ross authored a poem commemorating his achievement. It ended with:

> *O Death, where is thy sting?*
> *Thy victory, O Grave?*
> *First Corinthians 15:55 (KVJ)*

See the section on Malaria.

1905 – Smallpox and the Supreme Court

The U.S. Supreme Court upheld the constitutionality of mandatory smallpox vaccination programs when an epidemic endangers a community's population.

> *In every well-ordered society charged with the duty of conserving the safety of its members, the rights of the individual in respect of his liberty may at times, under the pressure of great dangers, be subjected to such restraint to be enforced by reasonable regulations, as the safety of the general public may demand.*
> *Jacobson v. Massachusetts*

1906 – A Test for Syphilis

German bacteriologist August Paul von Wassermann (1866–1925) invented a complement fixation test for syphilis. The Wassermann test detected syphilis early and could help prevent syphilis transmission.

1907 – Nobel Prize for Malaria Research

Charles Louis Alphonse Laveran received the Nobel Prize for discovering that the cause of Malaria is the protozoan *Plasmodium*. He also found the protozoan that causes African Sleeping Sickness.

1907 – Typhoid Mary

New Yorker Mary Mallon worked as a cook for a family that contracted typhoid fever. Health officials discovered that other families she worked for had contracted the same disease. They found that Mallon carried typhoid bacteria and was immune, but she could spread it to others. A judge confined her to a hospital for three years. She was released in 1910 and promised not to work as a cook, but she did and infected twenty-five people in 1915, one of whom died. After that, Mallon stayed in hospitals until she died in 1938. Typhoid Mary caused ten outbreaks, fifty-one cases of typhoid fever, and three deaths.

1916 – Measles in America

Twelve thousand people died in the epidemic. Seventy-five percent were under the age of five years.

1916 – Polio in America

The epidemic killed six thousand people and paralyzed thousands more for life.

1918 – The Great Flu Pandemic

From March 1918 to June 1920, the Spanish Flu spread to every part of the world, even the Arctic and remote Pacific islands. The first wave, in early March, resembled the typical flu. However, by August, the virus had mutated into a much deadlier form, and its victims were healthy young adults.

This deadly pandemic may have killed more people than the Black Death. One-third of the world's population was infected. At least fifty million people died worldwide—most within six months. Seventeen million died in India, which was five percent of the total population. In Japan, 390,000 people perished. In the U.S., the flu killed approximately 500,000 people. In Britain, 250,000 died. In France, 400,000 lost their lives. Native villages in Alaska were utterly wiped out.

Symptoms were unusual, and the Spanish flu was often misdiagnosed as dengue, cholera, or typhoid. Complications included bleeding from the nose, stomach, intestines, and ears. Death resulted from massive hemorrhage and lung edema.

In 1933, the influenza A virus was isolated. A vaccine became available in 1944, and by 1950, vaccination had become routine.

In 1998, Johan Hultin recovered DNA samples from a Native Alaskan woman's frozen corpse buried in permafrost for eighty years. Researchers analyzed the genetic structure of the 1918 virus. In 2000, Sir John Skehel and Professor Ian Wilson synthesized the hemagglutinin protein, which is responsible for its lethality. In 2005, researchers at the Mount Sinai School of Medicine in New York completely reconstructed the genetic sequence of the 1918 influenza. It was a subtype of avian H1N1.

1920 – Creutzfeldt-Jakob Disease

In 1920, German neurologists Hans Gerhard Creutzfeldt and Alfons Maria Jakob described cases of Creutzfeldt–Jakob disease. By 1997, over 100 cases of transmissible CJD had been reported, and new cases continued to emerge. CJD is a transmissible spongiform encephalopathy (TSE) caused by prions. Prions are misfolded proteins in the neurons of the central nervous system (CNS). They impair signaling, damage neurons, and create the spongiform appearance in the affected brain. The CJD prion induces the native prion protein to refold into a diseased form. The number of misfolded protein molecules increases exponentially, leading to a substantial accumulation of insoluble protein in affected cells. The accumulation of misfolded proteins disrupts neuronal cell function and ultimately leads to cell death.

1921 – Diphtheria in America

There were 206,000 cases of Diphtheria and 15,520 deaths.

1921 – Polio and FDR

Franklin Delano Roosevelt (1882–1945), former New York State Senator, Assistant Secretary to the Navy, and future U.S. president, contracted Polio. It paralyzed both his legs. The newspapers never photographed him in a wheelchair or using crutches.

1921 – Vaccine vs. Tuberculosis

French physician and bacteriologist Albert Calmette and veterinarian Camille Guérin noticed that a glycerin-bile-potato mixture grew less virulent tuberculosis bacilli. For the next thirteen years, even during World War I, these two incredibly persistent scientists recultured their tame TB bacillus 239 times and finally isolated a completely non-virulent strain in 1921, which enabled the production of the BCG vaccine.

Today, most countries use the BCG vaccine. However, the United States relies on testing to detect TB instead of vaccinating against it because the disease is now rare in the U.S.

1923 – Vaccine vs. Diphtheria

Vaccination decreased Diphtheria worldwide by 90% from 1980 to 2000. About 86% of the world's population is now immune.

1925 to 1950

The world's population was 2.5 billion. The average worldwide Life expectancy at birth in industrialized countries was fifty years.

1925 – Smallpox in Milwaukee

There were 386 cases and eighty-seven deaths. Three hundred twenty-seven of the victims were unvaccinated.

January 22, 1925 – The Alaskan Serum Run

An epidemic of Diphtheria is almost inevitable. I am in urgent need of one million units of diphtheria antitoxin. Mail is the only form of transportation.
Curtis Welch, MD – Radio message

When a child in Nome, Alaska, died, Dr. Welch diagnosed Diphtheria. Diphtheria attacks the nervous system and causes rapid death. It is highly contagious, with a fatality rate of ten percent among the general population and twenty percent in young children. Nome had 1300 settlers, and its only doctor could expect at least 200 deaths; all would be among his family and friends. The native population around Nome was 10,000, with no resistance to Diphtheria. Their mortality rate could approach 100%.

The only treatment was diphtheria antitoxin, but Dr. Welch's supply had expired, so he radioed for help. Planes couldn't fly in the icy winter, and there was no way by sea. The serum would have to come by sled dogs from Tanana,

674 miles away, across a harsh landscape in a blizzard with temperatures of minus 60 degrees.

Wild Bill Shannon left Tanana with the serum and made it to Minto, freezing and frostbitten. After replacing his dog team, he mushed to Tolovana, and Edgar Kalland took over. Kalland carried the serum to Bishop Mountain. The temperature was 62 below zero and dropping. From Bishop Mountain to Nulato, Charlie Evans's two lead dogs froze to death. Still, he managed to carry the serum to Tommy Patsey. Then Victor Anagick passed it to Myles Gonangnan at Unalakleet. The wind chill was 70 below zero with gale-force winds, but Gonangnan made it to Shaktoolik.

Henry Ivanoff took the serum and headed into the blizzard. Leonhard Seppala went to meet him. Pushing south from Nome, he met Ivanoff outside Shaktoolik, transferred the serum, and carried it back to Nome — covering eighty-four miles in 24 hours and climbing over Little McKinley Mountain twice, five thousand feet, each way! At Gloving, he passed the serum to Charlie Olsen. Olsen suffered from frostbite but made it to Bluff, where Gunnar Kassen and his dog, Balto, waited.

Kassen and Balto braved a sixty-mile-per-hour headwind in a whiteout blizzard. When his sled overturned, Kassen froze his hands, digging the precious antitoxin out of the snow. He made Point Safety ahead of schedule, but Ed Rohn was not ready, so Kassen continued! Gunnar Kassen and Balto covered the last twenty-five miles to Nome in just two hours. The teams covered 674 miles in 127.5 hours and stopped the epidemic.

Every year, there is an Iditarod dog sled race in Alaska. However, it is doubtful that any team of men and dogs could ever surpass the effort put forth in five days in 1925.

In 1995, Universal Pictures released the animated film *Balto*. There is a bronze statue of Balto in New York's Central Park.

1926 – Vaccine vs. Pertussis

Pediatrician Leila Denmark produced the first vaccine against pertussis (whooping cough) using killed *Bordetella pertussis* bacteria. Researchers developed acellular pertussis vaccines in the 1980s.

1927 – Malaria vs. Syphilis

Dementia paralytica, also known as general paralysis of the insane (GPI) or paralytic dementia, is caused by late-stage neurosyphilis. Victims develop dementia and have delusions of immense wealth. They talk incessantly, become violent, and finally die in a coma. Before penicillin, GPI was fatal and responsible for 25% of admissions to psychiatric hospitals. GPI killed Lord Randolph Churchill, Schumann, Donizetti, and Guy de Maupassant. Careful reading reveals GPI symptoms in the fictional characters created by authors such as Sir Arthur Conan Doyle, Agatha Christie, and Jack London, among others.

Julius Wagner-Jauregg transfused blood directly from patients with Malaria to patients with GPI. The resulting high fevers killed spirochetes and stopped the progression of GPI. After four bouts of high fever, quinine cured malaria-infected patients. Julius Wagner-Jauregg received the Nobel Prize for using Malaria to treat dementia paralytica.

1928 – Vaccinia Virus Grown in Lab

In 1928, H. B. Maitland and M. C. Maitland grew the vaccinia virus in minced hens' kidneys.

1930 – Vaccine vs. Yellow Fever

Yellow fever began in Africa. Then, the virus and its mosquito vector, A. Aegyptus, came on ships, bringing enslaved captives to the western hemisphere. The first outbreak of yellow fever on the North American continent was in 1647 in Barbados, followed by another in 1648 in Yucatan.

Yellow fever erupted in New York in 1668. In 1793, yellow fever killed 9% of Philadelphia's population. Epidemics of yellow fever swept through the Americas, and outbreaks even reached southern Europe. The last epidemic in the U.S. occurred in 1905 in New Orleans. In Cuba, Carlos Finlay proposed in 1881 that mosquitoes spread yellow fever. Army doctors, led by the physician Walter Reed, proved Finlay correct. William Gorgas conquered yellow fever in Havana and fought it in Panama.

In 1930, Max Theiler developed two vaccines against Yellow Fever. He won the Nobel Prize in 1951.

1931 – Influenza Virus Cultured

American pathologists Ernest William Goodpasture and Alice Miles Woodruff grew the influenza virus in fertilized chicken eggs.

1935 – Rats, Lice, and History

Hans Zinsser received his undergraduate degree from Columbia University in 1899. He completed his master's degree and a doctorate in medicine in 1903. Zinsser became an associate professor at Stanford University in 1910 and taught at Harvard Medical School. His specialties were bacteriology and immunology.

Himself a victim of typhus, Zinsser became an authority in the field, contributing to research that led to the mass production of rickettsia for study. He isolated the bacterium and developed a vaccine.

In 1935, he wrote the brilliant and original *Rats, Lice, and History, A Biography of Typhus*, tracing the vermin-borne disease's effects on armies, cities, and populations.

1936 – Another Yellow Fever Vaccine

Max Theiler and colleagues developed a better vaccine for Yellow Fever.

1938 – The March of Dimes

On his radio show, *The March of Time*, Eddie Cantor suggested sending dimes to President Roosevelt to fight Polio. Within weeks, 2,680,000 dimes arrived at the White House, prompting Franklin D. Roosevelt to establish the *March of Dimes*. Cities set up booths every Christmas season where children can insert their dimes into a slot. Seven billion dimes went to the war on Polio. A grateful nation minted the Roosevelt dime in the President's honor.

1939 – DDT

Paul Müller discovered DDT's insecticidal properties in 1939. In World War II, DDT controlled Malaria and typhus and saved countless lives. After the war, DDT boosted agricultural productivity. Müller received the 1948 Nobel Prize in Medicine for his discovery of the effectiveness of DDT against arthropods.

1941 – Rubella Causes Congenital Defects

Australian ophthalmologist Norman McAlister Gregg linked rubella during pregnancy to the development of congenital cataracts. It gradually became clear that rubella in the first trimester causes congenital disabilities. Two-thirds of babies were blind, had heart and neurological abnormalities, and were deaf.

1941 – Vaccine vs. Tick-Borne Encephalitis

TBE is a viral disease transmitted by arthropods that is endemic to most European countries. Scientists developed the first vaccine in 1941, followed by an inactivated virus vaccine. Outbreaks of TBE involving thousands of cases still occur.

1945 – Vaccine vs. Influenza

An influenza vaccine became a priority for the U.S. military after one in every sixty American soldiers died during the Spanish Flu Pandemic. The first vaccine was an inactivated subtype of the influenza A virus. Then, researchers discovered influenza type B, the leading cause of seasonal epidemics. A whole-virus inactivated influenza A and B vaccine began military use in the United States in 1945 and civilian use in 1946. The key investigators were Thomas Francis Jr., MD, and Jonas Salk, MD. They later worked on the polio vaccine.

July 28, 1945 – The First AIDS Death?

Sadayo Fujisawa of Montreal, Canada, died of cytomegalovirus, diarrhea, and an unknown "wasting disease." However, retrospective analysis suggests that she died of AIDS.

1946 – Streptomycin versus Tuberculosis

Selman Abraham Waksman discovered streptomycin, the first antibiotic to treat tuberculosis.

1947–1951 – Malaria Eliminated from America

In 1947, there were 15,000 cases of malaria in America. The United States National Malaria Eradication Program was established in the same year. By 1949, it had sprayed 4,650,000 houses, inside and out, with DDT. By 1950, the number of malaria infections had dropped to just 2,000.

In 1951, the CDC shifted the program to focus solely on surveillance, and in 1952, the malaria program was discontinued.

My father, James Hollis Jones, contracted malaria during World War II. He experienced several recurrences in the 1950s after his return from China and Africa.

1947 – Zika Virus

Researchers found a new virus among rhesus monkeys living in the Zika forest in Uganda.

1947 – Smallpox in New York City

Eugene Le Bar was ill when he arrived in New York from Mexico City. He went to a hospital, where he died of smallpox. The infection spread to two other patients who were also in the hospital at the same time. Health Commissioner Israel Weinstein oversaw the vaccination of 6.35 million people, limiting the epidemic to only ten additional cases and one more death.

1949 – Polio Virus Cultured

John Franklin Enders, Thomas Weller, and Frederick Robbins grew poliovirus in human embryo cells. Later, Jonas Salk used the process to make the polio vaccine.

1950 to 1960

The world's population was three billion.

1950 – Kuru

Kuru is a rare, incurable, and invariably fatal neurodegenerative disorder formerly common among the Fore people of Papua New Guinea. In reports, Australian officers patrolling the Eastern Highlands of Papua New Guinea first described Kuru in the early 1950s. Kuru is a form of transmissible spongiform encephalopathy (TSE) caused by abnormally folded proteins (prions), which leads to tremors and loss of coordination from neurodegeneration.

The infectious agent is a misfolded form of a host-encoded protein called prion (PrP). Prion proteins are encoded by the Prion Protein Gene (PRNP)

Australian Michael Alpers conducted extensive field studies among the Fore with Shirley Lindenbaum. Their research suggested the epidemic originated in 1900 from a single individual who spontaneously developed Creutzfeldt–Jakob disease.

Kuru spread easily and rapidly due to funeral practices in which relatives consumed the corpses of family members after they had been buried for days and colonized by insect larvae. The disinterred corpse was then dismembered and served with the larvae as a side dish.

With the banning of cannibalism by Australian colonial law enforcement and local missionaries' efforts, kuru was declining by the mid-1960s — the last person known to have had kuru died in 2009.

1950 – Prions

In the 1950s, Carleton Gajdusek proved that kuru could be transmitted to chimpanzees by a new infectious agent (a prion). He won the 1976 Nobel Prize for medicine.

1951 – Influenza Hits England and Canada

Influenza caused an unusual number of deaths in England and Canada. In some areas, it was even higher than in the 1918 pandemic.

1952 – Nobel Prize for Streptomycin

The Prize went to Selman Abraham Waksman for the discovery of streptomycin, the first antibiotic effective against tuberculosis.

1952 – Polio in America

In 1952 and 1953, America had 93,000 polio cases, a massive increase from the earlier average of 20,000 a year. Many victims lived out their lives in Iron Lungs. I had schoolmates with polio-withered arms and legs.

1952 – Salk, Sabin, and the Polio Vaccine

Millions of dollars were spent to find a polio vaccine. Jonas Salk developed an inactivated poliovirus vaccine in 1952. Clinical trials began in 1954 with 20,000 physicians,

64,000 school personnel, 220,000 volunteers, and 1.8 million school children. The successful test led to widespread vaccinations.

My father, James Hollis Jones, MD, had seen Polio paralyze his brother. I was six, but I still remember his excitement when the Salk vaccine arrived at his office. After dinner, he drove our family to his office to get the shot. He did the same when Albert Sabin developed the live oral vaccine in 1962.

The last outbreak of paralytic poliomyelitis in the United States was in 1979 among unvaccinated Amish. Polio disappeared from the Americas by 1994 and from 36 Western Pacific countries, including China and Australia, by 2000. Europe was polio-free in 2002. Worldwide, polio cases dropped from 350,000 in 1988 to 1,300 in 2007. By 2008, Polio remained only in Nigeria, India, Pakistan, and Afghanistan. In 2016, there were only five cases of wild poliovirus in Pakistan and one in Afghanistan. Polio eradication efforts stalled in 2019 due to wars, politics, and vaccine hesitancy.

1952 – Isoniazid for Tuberculosis

Isoniazid, also known as isonicotinylhydrazide (INH), was tested in Navajo communities to treat tuberculosis. With isoniazid, a cure for TB is possible.

1954 – Vaccine vs. Anthrax

Austrian-South African immunologist Max Sterne (1905–1997) developed an attenuated live animal vaccine in 1935. The "Sterne strain" of anthrax forms the basis of livestock anthrax vaccines worldwide. A British anthrax vaccine became available for human use in 1954.

1956–1958 – The Asian Flu Pandemic

The Asian flu originated in Guizhou, China, in 1956. It was an H2N2 subtype with avian influenza virus RNA. It spread to Singapore, Hong Kong, and worldwide, killing two million people. In 1968, it mutated to H3N2 and triggered another pandemic.

1957 – Vaccine vs. Adenovirus

Adenovirus vaccines first appeared in the 1950s. By 1960, a live-virus vaccine effective against serotype 4 disease was available for military use. Vaccines for types 4 and 7 became standard for military trainees in 1971. The vaccine significantly decreased disease rates by 95%. In 1994, the manufacturer announced it would stop producing the vaccines. Physicians administered the last doses in 1995.

1958 – Burkett's Lymphoma

Burkett, D., A sarcoma involving the jaws in African children, Brit. J. Surg., 1958, 46:218-23.

The geographic spread of this African cancer suggested that a vector was responsible. It provided the first evidence that viruses can cause cancer. Research led to the discovery of the Epstein-Barr Virus.

1959 – HIV in Humans

Researchers believe that, in the 1900s, the Simian immunodeficiency virus infected humans in central Africa. As a result, it became the HIV pandemic.

A preserved blood sample proved that a human death from HIV occurred in the Congo in 1959. On June 28, 1959, Ardouin Antonio, a 49-year-old Haitian, died in New York City of Pneumocystis jirovecii disease secondary to AIDS.

1960 to 1970

The world's population was 3.7 billion.

Coronaviruses

Virologists isolated Coronaviruses in the 1960s. They cause colds, pneumonia, diarrhea, and bronchitis in chickens, pigs, cows, cats, dogs, civets, ferrets, mice, camels, and bats.

Coronaviruses have jumped from animals to humans three times:

From 2002 to 2004, SARS-CoV caused an epidemic of *Severe Acute Respiratory Syndrome* (**SARS**). Over 8,000 people were infected, and 10 percent died.

In 2012, the Coronavirus MERS-CoV caused *Middle East Respiratory Syndrome.* In 2013, there were 124 cases in Saudi Arabia, with fifty-two deaths. In 2015, the epidemic reached Korea, and by 2019, 2468 cases of **MERS** had killed 851, a mortality rate of 35%. Sporadic cases of MERS continue to occur.

In December 2019, the **COVID-19** pandemic (caused by the Coronavirus SARS-CoV-2)began in China and spread worldwide. Coronavirus 229E, coronavirus OC43, coronavirus NL63, and coronavirus HKU1 infect humans, but as of 2021, they have not yet caused epidemics.

1961–1975 – Seventh Cholera Pandemic

Once again, Cholera spread from Indonesia to Bangladesh, India, the Soviet Union, Italy, Japan, and the South Pacific. Deaths were low because of modern medicine. In 1991, the same strain surfaced in Peru, killing 10,000.

1963 – Vaccine vs. Measles

Twenty years after being licensed in the U.S., measles vaccination prevented 52 million cases of the disease, 17,400 cases of brain damage, and 5,200 deaths. Worldwide, the measles vaccine saved 1.4 million lives.

1964 – Rubella in America

Rubella afflicted 12.5 million people in the U.S. and caused 2,000 deaths. In addition, it infected 50,000 vulnerable pregnant women, causing thousands of miscarriages. Sadly, 20,000 children were born with the horrible congenital rubella syndrome, 8,000 were born deaf, and 3,500 were born deaf and blind.

The Australian Antigen

In 1964, Baruch Blumberg discovered an antigen in the blood of an Australian Aboriginal person. Initially, he thought it was a genetic marker of prehistoric migrations. However, in 1968, virologist Alfred Prince proved the antigen was the Hepatitis B Virus. Blumberg developed a screening test for hepatitis B and showed that the virus caused liver cancer. He developed a vaccine and distributed the patent for free.

The vaccine reduced childhood Hepatitis B cases in China from 15% to 1% over 10 years. Blumberg received the 1976 Nobel Prize for discoveries related to new mechanisms for the origin and spread of infectious diseases.

1965 – Retroviruses Discovered

Howard Temin described the first retrovirus.

1967 – Vaccine vs. Mumps

The U.S. FDA approved a vaccine developed by Maurice Hilleman from the mumps virus he collected from his five-year-old daughter, Jeryl Lynn Hilleman. It was in routine use by 1977.

1967 – Zombie Deer Disease

Chronic wasting disease (CWD) is a prion disease causing transmissible spongiform encephalopathy (TSE) in free-ranging and farmed deer, elk, caribou, moose, and reindeer. It was first documented in the U.S. in 1967. Prions cause fatal neurodegenerative diseases in humans and animals by converting the cellular prion protein PrPC into aggregation-prone PrPSc, similar to TSEs like mad cow disease, Creutzfeldt-Jakob disease, and scrapie.

Animals infected with CWD show abnormal behavior in the later stages, including stumbling, drooling, and acting strangely. CWD is always fatal, and currently, there is no known cure or vaccine. The cause of CWD is prions, abnormal proteins that are highly resistant to eradication. Disinfectants and high heat cannot destroy prions.

CWD is highly contagious and spreads through contact between animals and contact with prions in manure-contaminated environments, where prions can persist for decades. The disease is rapidly spreading in wild and captive animals across 30 U.S. states and four Canadian provinces. CWD has also infected wild reindeer in Norway and moose in Finland, Sweden, and South Korea.

Although no link has yet been established between CWD and human TSE, hunters should minimize their risk by avoiding handling or eating meat from animals that appear sick, behave strangely, or are found dead. Wear latex or nitrile gloves when butchering animals, and avoid contact with organs—especially the brain and spinal cord. Test all deer and elk for CWD before consuming any meat.

1968 – The Hong Kong Flu Pandemic

The 1968 influenza pandemic first appeared in Hong Kong and subsequently spread across Asia. It affected India, the Philippines, Australia, and Europe. American soldiers returning from Vietnam brought it to California. By 1969, it had reached Japan, Africa, and South America. It resurfaced in 1969, 1970, and 1972.

In 1972, I caught the Hong Kong Flu while working as an intern at John Gaston Hospital in Memphis. I experienced bone-chilling chills, high fevers, intense muscle pain, and coughed up Curschmann's spirals. A 50-year-old smoker likely would have died. It truly scared me. Since then, I get the influenza vaccine every year. I never want to be that sick again.

1970 to 1980

The world's population was 4.3 billion.

1970 – Vaccine vs. Rubella

In 1964, at the Wistar Institute, Stanley Plotkin developed the rubella vaccine, which is now used worldwide. He also co-invented the rotavirus vaccine.

1972 – Smallpox in Yugoslavia

The last European outbreak of smallpox was in 1972 in Yugoslavia.

1974 – Vaccine vs. Chickenpox

Takahashi's 1974 discovery of the attenuation of the varicella-zoster virus led to the development of a live chickenpox vaccine, resulting in a significant reduction in hospitalizations and deaths. A more potent version of the vaccine now protects against herpes zoster.

1975 – The End of Variola Major

The last case of the deadly Variola major smallpox occurred in Bangladesh in October 1975.

1975 – Hepatitis C

Harvey J. Alter discovered that post-transfusion hepatitis cases were not caused by hepatitis A or B. However, it took twelve years to identify the cause of non-A, non-B hepatitis. Finally, in 1987, Michael Houghton, Qui-Lim Choo, and

George Kuo used molecular cloning to find the virus and develop a diagnostic test. Screening reduced the risk of blood transfusion hepatitis to zero.

1976 – Ebola Hemorrhagic Fever

The disease emerged in 1976 during simultaneous outbreaks, one in Nzara and the other in Yambuku, villages near the Ebola River. It is a viral hemorrhagic fever that affects humans and primates. The initial symptoms include fever, sore throat, muscle pain, and headache. Vomiting, diarrhea, and a skin rash soon develop, followed by severe damage to the liver and kidneys. Ultimately, victims bleed internally and externally. The disease has a fifty percent case fatality rate.

1977 – Patient Zero

A study in *The American Journal of Medicine* traced many HIV infections to male flight attendant French-Canadian Gaëtan Dugas. Dugas had 2,500 sexual partners across North America. He was part of a cluster of gay men who traveled often, were sexually active, and all died of AIDS early in the epidemic.

1977 – Streptococcus Pneumonia Vaccine

The United States approved the first polysaccharide pneumococcal vaccine in 1977. It contained antigens from fourteen different pneumococcal bacteria. In 1983, a 23-valent polysaccharide vaccine replaced the 14-valent vaccine.

1977 – The End of Variola Minor

The last recorded case of Variola minor (smallpox) occurred in Merca, Somalia, in October 1977. It was the final smallpox case on Earth.

1978 – Vaccine vs. Meningitis

Meningococcal deaths declined after the discovery of sulfonamides, but sulfa-resistant strains infected new military recruits.

The U.S. military developed an A-polysaccharide vaccine in 1968. Military scientists also produced a meningococcal serogroup A polysaccharide vaccine. By 1971, all new U.S. recruits received the meningococcal serogroup C vaccine. In 1974, the FDA licensed meningococcal polysaccharide vaccines for civilian use.

1980 to 1990

The world population was 5.2 billion.

1980 – The Extinction of Smallpox

In 1980, the World Health Organization declared smallpox extinct. The virus still exists at the Centers for Disease Control and Prevention in the United States and the State Center for Research on Virology and Biotechnology in Novosibirsk, Russia. For the first time in history, humans defeated a disease.

1981 – HIV/AIDS

On June 5, 1981, the U.S. Centers for Disease Control recorded a cluster of Pneumocystis carinii pneumonia in five gay men in Los Angeles. The AIDS pandemic began eighty years after the simian immunodeficiency virus crossed over to humans in central Africa.

HIV spread from Africa to Haiti and entered the United States in 1969. By 2007, over thirty million people had HIV, and 2.1 million died that year.

1981 – Vaccine vs. Hepatitis B

The hepatitis B vaccine was the first vaccine to target a cause of cancer.

1982 – Prions isolated

In 1982, Stanley B. Prusiner announced that his team had purified an "infectious protein," which was not present in healthy hosts. He named the protein "prion" for "proteinaceous infectious particle." After discovering the same protein in a different form in uninfected individuals, the prion protein was named PrP. Griffith correctly hypothesized that the abnormal protein converts normal proteins of its type into the abnormal form. Prusiner won the Nobel Prize in Physiology or Medicine in 1997 for his research into prions.

1982 – Helicobacter Pylori

Marshall and Warren hypothesized that bacteria caused peptic ulcers and gastric cancer. In 1984, Marshall proved that Helicobacter pylori caused gastritis by using himself as a test subject. First, he was gastroscoped, and no H. pylori was present. However, after swallowing H. pylori, he developed gastritis. A second gastroscopy found the organism. He took antibiotics and soon became asymptomatic. A third gastroscopy did not detect any H. pylori.

Marshall discovered that antibiotics used to treat H. pylori also healed ulcers and some stomach cancers. In 2005, Barry J. Marshall and J. Robin Warren received the Nobel Prize.

1983 – HIV Virus Identified

Luc Montagnier at the Pasteur Institute in France isolated the HIV retrovirus.

1985 – Vaccine vs. Haemophilus Influenzae

Before the vaccine, Haemophilus influenzae was a leading cause of childhood meningitis, pneumonia, and epiglottitis in the United States, causing 20,000 cases annually in the 1980s, mostly in children under five. Since the introduction of routine vaccination, the disease has decreased by 99%. As a result, Haemophilus influenzae went from infecting one hundred children out of every 100,000 to fewer than one per 100,000. It was no longer a public health concern. Similar results occurred in Western Europe and developing countries.

1986–2001 – Mad Cow and Creutzfeldt–Jakob Disease

In the 1980s, it was a widespread practice in industrialized countries to feed young calves grain mixed with ground-up meat and bones from the unusable parts of dead cattle. Unfortunately, some diseased cattle brains contained a prion — it spread to the calves that ate the mixture. As a result, Bovine spongiform encephalopathy erupted in the UK. It infected 231 humans, causing Creutzfeldt–Jakob disease. The UK eradication program culled 4 million cows, and countries regulated animal feed contents. By 2017, there were only four cases worldwide.

1987 – Antiretroviral HIV Therapy

The FDA approved zidovudine (AZT) for HIV in 1987. More NRTIs followed, but patients still died. Finally, in 1996, Hammer and Gulick demonstrated the benefit of combining two NRTIs with protease inhibitors. Three-drug therapy led to a sixty percent reduction in HIV deaths.

1989–2020 – RNA Vaccines

In 1989, researchers at the Salk Institute, University of California, San Diego, and Vical Incorporated used a liposomal nanoparticle to deliver mRNA into different cells.

In 1990, Jon A. Wolff showed that mRNA injected into mice delivered the genetic information to produce proteins within living cell tissue.

In 1993, Martinon demonstrated that liposome-encapsulated RNA activated T-cells. Then, in 1994, Zhou & Berglund presented evidence that RNA could serve as a vaccine.

An mRNA vaccine "transfects" synthetic RNA into human cells, directing them to produce the foreign protein typically made by the virus. The protein triggers an immune response that destroys any invading virus with a protein that is identical to it. As a result, RNA vaccines are quicker to develop and less expensive to produce.

Hungarian biochemists Katalin Kariko and Drew Weissman solved technical barriers to getting mRNA inside human cells without setting off the body's defense system.

In 2005, Derrick Rossi founded the mRNA-focused biotech Moderna with Robert Langer.

In 2020, Moderna and Pfizer/BioNTech developed mRNA-based COVID-19 vaccines funded by Operation Warp Speed.

1990 to 2000

The world's population was six billion.

1991 – Cholera in South America

More than one million people were infected, with 10,000 deaths.

1991 – Magic Johnson has HIV

On November 7, 1991, Earvin "Magic" Johnson Jr. announced he had HIV. However, he said that his wife and unborn child did not have it and would dedicate his life to defeating his disease. In 2022, Magic Johnson was alive and well. He is proof of HIV medications' effectiveness and the importance of adhering to medical treatment.

1991 – Vaccine vs. Hepatitis A

The vaccine prevents hepatitis A, is effective in 95% of patients, and provides protection for at least 15 years.

1993 – Cryptosporidium in Milwaukee

In 1993, the chlorine-resistant parasite *Cryptosporidium parvum* invaded the Milwaukee water supply. It infected 400,000 people and cost $96 million.

1994 – Black Death Returns to India

Bubonic and Pneumonic Plague infected 693 and killed fifty-six.

1995 – HIV Protease Inhibitor

Saquinavir, a protease inhibitor, was approved to treat HIV. As a result, highly Active Antiretroviral Therapy (HAART) began, and AIDS death rates plummeted.

1995 –Prion Surveillance Center

The National Prion Disease Pathology Surveillance Center (NPDPSC) was established in 1997 in the "Division of Neuropathology" at Case Western Reserve University by Dr. Pierluigi Gambetti. It is the only Center of its kind in the U.S. The NPDPSC coordinates autopsies and collects tissue samples and clinical information from cases of prion disease to assist the Centers for Disease Control and Prevention (CDC) in determining the disease's incidence and investigating cases of possible transmission from other humans or animals (such as chronic wasting disease, possibly transmitting from deer to humans). The Center operates the nation's clinical reference lab for prion disease and performs cerebrospinal fluid and genetic testing. They offer a brain MRI consultation program.

1998 –The MMR Vaccine Hoax

The most damaging medical hoax
of the last one hundred years.
Dennis K Flaherty

In 1998, The Lancet published a flawed research paper. It falsely reported that the measles, mumps, and rubella vaccine (MMR) caused autism. Unfortunately, widespread media coverage was naive and lent credibility to these false claims. As a result, vaccination rates dropped sharply, and cases of measles and mumps increased significantly. In the following decades, many deaths and permanent disabilities occurred.

The paper's author had conflicts of interest, manipulated evidence, and violated ethical codes. As a result, the Lancet retracted the article in 2010. The Lancet's editor-in-chief described it as *"utterly false"* and said the journal had been *"deceived."* The General Medical Council of the United Kingdom found Wakefield guilty of serious professional misconduct in May 2010. As a result, he can no longer practice in the U.K. In 2011, the British Medical Journal labeled his paper as fraudulent.

Investigations by journalist Brian Deer for *The Sunday Times*, and later confirmed by the *British Medical Journal* (BMJ), uncovered that Wakefield was paid to find scientific evidence that could support claims against the MMR vaccine. Wakefield received the money over several years, beginning well before the publication of his 1998 *Lancet* paper that falsely linked the MMR vaccine to autism. He did not disclose this financial conflict of interest to *The Lancet* or to his fellow researchers, a serious breach of ethical standards.

Following years of investigation, the UK General Medical Council held disciplinary hearings and found Wakefield guilty of serious professional misconduct, including dishonesty, unethical treatment of children, and failure to disclose his financial ties to the anti-vaccine legal campaign. In 2010, he was struck off the UK medical register, permanently losing his license to practice medicine. That same year, *The Lancet* fully retracted his paper, calling its findings "utterly false."

Subsequent large-scale epidemiological studies involving millions of children around the world have shown no link between the MMR vaccine and autism. Wakefield's fraudulent work is now regarded as one of the most damaging and unethical acts in modern medical research, having fueled decades of vaccine hesitancy based on fabricated evidence.

Wakefield accepted undisclosed payments from lawyers preparing lawsuits against vaccine manufacturers before and during the time he conducted his faulty research on the MMR vaccine.

https://www.bmj.com/content/342/bmj.c5258?utm_source

https://www.bmj.com/content/342/bmj.c5347?utm_source

Following years of investigation, the UK General Medical Council held disciplinary hearings and found Wakefield guilty of serious professional misconduct, dishonesty, unethical treatment of children, and failure to disclose financial ties to the anti-vaccine legal campaign. In 2010, he was struck off the UK medical register, permanently losing his license to practice medicine. That same year, *The Lancet* fully retracted his paper, calling its findings "utterly false."

Subsequent large-scale epidemiological studies involving millions of children around the world have shown no link between the MMR vaccine and autism.

Wakefield's fraudulent work is now regarded as one of the most damaging and unethical acts in modern medical research, having fueled decades of vaccine hesitancy based on fabricated evidence.

Extensive epidemiological studies and reviews by the Institute of Medicine, the U.S. National Academy of

Sciences, the UK National Health Service, and the Cochrane Library found no link between MMR and autism.

The United States National Vaccine Injury Compensation Program rejected claims from parents of children with autism. The overwhelming scientific consensus is that the MMR vaccine has no link to the development of autism.

Measles, Mumps, Rubella Vaccination and Autism: A Nationwide Cohort Study (Hviid et al., 2019) – This Danish cohort study included 657,461 children born between 1999 and 2010. The fully adjusted hazard ratio comparing vaccinated versus unvaccinated children was 0.93 (95% CI: 0.85-1.02), indicating no increased risk of autism after MMR vaccination.

https://pubmed.ncbi.nlm.nih.gov/30831578/

Autism Occurrence by MMR Vaccine Status Among US Children With Older Siblings With and Without Autism (Kaiser Permanente/US cohort study) – This U.S.-based study examined children with older siblings who have ASD; even in that higher-risk group, they found no harmful link between MMR vaccination and autism.

https://jamanetwork.com/journals/jama/fullarticle/22 75444?utm_source=chatgpt.com

But the damage was already done, and its effects continued. For instance, a 2015 survey revealed that nine percent of Americans still wrongly believed the lie that the measles vaccine was harmful.

In 2016, an unrepentant Wakefield produced an anti-vaccination film alleging a conspiracy and cover-up by the U.S. Centers for Disease Control and Prevention.

1998 – Vaccine vs. Lyme Disease

The Lyme vaccine developed by SmithKline Beecham was 80% effective. Three FDA panel members mentioned a theoretical concern that the drug might cause autoimmune arthritis, which had not occurred in any clinical trial. Therefore, the panel unanimously approved the vaccine. Out of 1.4 million doses, only fifty-nine recipients reported arthritis – exactly the same rate as in unvaccinated individuals. The FDA found no link between the vaccine and arthritis.

However, it was the year of the MMR Vaccine Hoax, and people grew suspicious. The media covered every minor concern, and anti-vaccine groups pushed the Lyme vaccine off the market. As a result, no vaccine is available, and 30,000 Americans get Lyme disease each year.

1998 – Vaccine vs. Rotavirus

Rotavirus is the leading cause of severe diarrhea in children and infants worldwide. Before the vaccine's introduction, the disease resulted in 400,000 doctor visits and 200,000 emergency room visits annually in the United States. Wyeth Pharmaceuticals licensed RotaShield in 1998. Scientists linked the vaccine to a rare intestinal issue called intussusception, leading Wyeth to withdraw it. In 2006, H. Fred Clark, Ph.D., Stanley A. Plotkin, MD, and Paul A. Offit, MD, developed the RotaTeq vaccine. U.S. hospitalization rates for acute gastroenteritis decreased by sixteen percent in 2007 and by forty-five percent in 2008. Rotavirus kills 450,000 unvaccinated children under age five each year, with most deaths occurring in developing countries.

2000 to 2010

The world's population was seven billion.

2003 – Nasal Vaccine vs. Influenza

In 2003, the FDA approved FluMist, the first influenza vaccine delivered by a nasal spray. It uses a weakened live virus to induce immunity.

2003 – SARS Coronavirus Epidemic

The SARS-CoV Coronavirus causes Severe Acute Respiratory Syndrome. From 2002 to 2003, an outbreak in southern China spread worldwide to infect 8,098, with 774 deaths in thirty-seven countries and a ten percent fatality rate.

Carlo Urbani from Doctors Without Borders alerted the World Health Organization and initiated what became the most effective epidemic response in medical history. Sadly, Urbani himself contracted SARS and passed away.

There have been no SARS cases since 2004. However, in 2017, scientists traced the virus through civets to horseshoe bats in Yunnan province.

2005 – Nobel Prize for Helicobacter

Barry J. Marshall and J. Robin Warren received the Nobel Prize for discovering the bacterium Helicobacter pylori and its role in gastritis and peptic ulcer disease.

2005 – Dengue Fever in Singapore

Dengue infected 14,000, and twenty-seven people died

2005 – Chikungunya Pandemic

The Asian tiger mosquito and *Aedes aegypti* carry the Chikungunya virus. Outbreaks have spread around the world: 2005 in Réunion, then India, Thailand, the Pacific Islands, 2012 in Cambodia and the Caribbean, 2014 in the United States, Venezuela, France, Costa Rica, Brazil, El Salvador, 2014 in Mexico, Colombia, and 2019 Republic of the Congo.

2006 – Dengue in India and Pakistan

Dengue infected 3600 people in India and 2000 people in Pakistan. One hundred died.

2006 – Vaccine vs. Human Papillomavirus

The HPV vaccine prevents cervical, penile, and laryngeal cancer.

2007 – Zika Outbreak on the Island of Yap

Seventy percent of Yap Island residents contracted the Zika virus, first found in rhesus monkeys living in Uganda's Zika forest.

2007 – Cured of HIV

Timothy Ray Brown had leukemia and HIV. After receiving a bone marrow transplant from a homozygous CCR5-Δ32 donor, he recovered from both. However, the CCR5 receptor that his strain of HIV needed to enter cells was absent from his donor bone marrow.

Maraviroc is a CCR5 receptor antagonist used to treat AIDS.

2007 – Ebola in Africa

In August 2007, the Territoire de Mweka had an outbreak of Ebola, killing one hundred people.

2007 – Cholera in Iraq

Seven thousand were infected, with ten deaths.

2008 – Nobel Prize for HPV and HIV

Harald Zur Hausen received the prize for discovering that human papillomaviruses cause cervical cancer. Françoise Barré-Sinoussi and Luc Montagnier received it for isolating the human immunodeficiency virus.

2008 – Cholera in Zimbabwe

There were 98,000 cases of Cholera and 4,000 deaths

2009 – Dengue Fever in Bolivia

The worst outbreak of dengue fever in Bolivia's history killed eighteen out of 31,000 known victims.

2009 – Swine Flu Pandemic

From 2009 to 2010, approximately 11 percent of the world's population contracted the Swine Flu (H1N1), resulting in 150,000 deaths. The Swine Flu vaccine saved 300 lives and prevented one million illnesses in the U.S.

2010 to 2023

From 2010 to 2020, the world's population increased from 7 billion to 8 billion. The average life expectancy at birth in the USA is seventy-nine years. The global average is 72 years, with a range from 57 in Somalia to 85 in Japan.

2010 – Cholera in Haiti

Haiti's capital, Port-au-Prince, is one of the largest cities in the world without a sewage system. As a result, feces from three million people drain into canals and ditches, contaminating drinking water and spreading disease. No wonder that, after the 2010 earthquake, 4,787 Haitians died of cholera, which is now endemic across the country, infecting eight hundred thousand Haitians.

2011 – Dengue in Pakistan

Fourteen thousand were infected, and three hundred died.

2011 – The Extinction of Rinderpest

Rinderpest was an extremely contagious viral disease that infected cattle, domestic buffalo, large antelope, deer, giraffes, wildebeests, and warthogs, with death rates reaching nearly 100 percent. In June 2011, the United Nations confirmed that the disease is extinct. Rinderpest and smallpox are the only diseases in history to have been eradicated from the world.

2012 – Vaccine vs. Hepatitis E.

Scientists created a Hepatitis E vaccine in the 1990s, but production ceased due to lack of profitability. China still uses a vaccine developed by Chinese scientists in 2012. As of 2021, the United States does not have a licensed hepatitis E vaccine.

2012 – Quadrivalent influenza vaccine

2012 – MERS Coronavirus Epidemic

In September 2012, the *Middle East Respiratory Syndrome* (MERS) epidemic, caused by the Coronavirus MERS-CoV, began after the virus jumped from camels to humans. In 2013, there were 124 cases in Saudi Arabia, with fifty-two deaths; a year later, there were two cases in the United States. In 2015, the epidemic reached Korea. By 2019, 2,468 cases of MERS had killed 851 people, with a mortality rate of thirty-five percent. Sporadic cases continue to occur.

2012 – Yellow Fever in Sudan

Yellow fever broke out in Darfur, Sudan. There were 847 cases and 171 deaths.

2013 – Western African Ebola epidemic

The Western African Ebola epidemic (2013–2016) started in Guinea, Liberia, and Sierra Leone. It infected 28,616 people, killing 11,310. Survivors may have the post-Ebola syndrome and need care for years. Authorities have stockpiled 300,000 doses of the rVSV-ZEBOV vaccine for the next Ebola epidemic.

2013 – Treatment for Hepatitis C

Sofosbuvir inhibits the RNA polymerase that the Hepatitis C Virus uses to replicate. As a result, it has a high cure rate, few side effects, and a short duration of therapy.

2013 – Cholera in Cuba

The Cuban Health Ministry reported fifty-one cases.

2013 – Chikungunya in the Caribbean

The 2013–15 Caribbean Chikungunya epidemic spread quickly across the Caribbean. By 2014, there were approximately 355,000 cases.

2013–2016 - The Ebola Epidemic

The outbreak began in West Africa in 2013. There were 28,616 cases and 11,310 deaths.

2014 – Black Death in Madagascar

The Bubonic and pneumonic plague infected 119 victims and resulted in 40 deaths.

2015 – Nobel Prize for Parasites and Malaria

William C. Campbell and Satoshi Ōmura received the Nobel Prize for discovering a new therapy for infections caused by roundworm parasites. Youyou Tu received it for developing a new treatment for malaria.

2015 – Bat Coronaviruses Might Infect Humans

> *The emergence of SARS-CoV and MERS-CoV underscores the threat to humans. Our results indicate that coronavirus viruses encoding the SHC014 spike can replicate in humans. And that there is a potential risk of SARS-CoV re-emerging in the future.*
> *Nature Medicine VOLUME 21, NUMBER 12, DECEMBER 2015*
> *Vineet D Menachery, Boyd L Yount Jr, et al.*

2015 – Vaccine vs. Hand-Foot-Mouth Disease

Enterovirus 71 (EV-A71) causes hand, foot, and mouth epidemics in infants and young children. It is a severe problem in Asia and the Pacific, where EV-A71 infection often results in severe neurological complications and death. In 2015, China introduced the first vaccine against EV-A71.

2015 – CRISPR/Cas9 vs. HIV

Using CRISPR/Cas9 to inactivate HIV-1 Proviral DNA: Retrovirology 201512:22, article by Zhu, Lei, Le Duff, Li, Guo, Wainberg, and Liang

May 2015 – Zika in Brazil

In 2015, a Zika epidemic began in Brazil and spread throughout the Americas, the Pacific, and Asia. When Zika infects pregnant women, the baby is born with microcephaly, brain deformities, and neurological problems. To stop Zika, Brazil released genetically modified mosquitoes and reduced the *Aedes Aegypti* population by 90%.

2015 – Swine Flu Returns to India

There were 33,000 cases and 2,000 deaths.

2015 – Vaccine vs. Dengue fever

Dengue infects 400 million people annually. It is endemic in American Samoa, Guam, Puerto Rico, and the U.S. Virgin Islands. Severe cases can be fatal, especially among children.

The mosquito-borne Dengue virus is a single positive-sense RNA virus with four serotypes and forty-seven strains, all capable of causing the disease. The immune system produces antibodies and immunity specific to one serotype.

However, these antibodies do not neutralize other serotypes. As a result, reinfection with a different serotype leads to increased viral replication and can cause Hemorrhagic Fever and Dengue Shock Syndrome. Vaccination targeting only one serotype can also result in hemorrhagic fever and Dengue Shock if the person is infected with another serotype. Therefore, an ideal vaccine must protect against all four serotypes.

The vaccine, Dengvaxia, prevents all dengue serotype infections in people who _previously had dengue_. However, it increases the severity of the disease in people not previously infected.

2015 – CRISPR-Cas9 and Mosquitos

A biotech company developed Aedes aegypti mosquitoes with a self-limiting gene that causes their offspring to die. They also have a fluorescent marker for easy identification. The mosquitoes were released in Piracicaba, Brazil, from 2015 until mid-2016. This led to a reduction in dengue cases from 133 to twelve.

2016 – Zika in America

The virus entered northeastern Brazil in 2013, thriving in areas with dense populations and hordes of Aedes aegypti mosquitoes — circulating a year before being detected in 2015. By 2016, 2000 babies in Brazil were born with Zika-related microcephaly. In 2014, Zika reached the Caribbean, and Infected mosquitoes hitchhiked on cruise ships and planes to Miami. In 2016, Florida reported 256 cases of Zika.

2016 – Yellow Fever in Angola and the Congo

500 people died.

2016–2019 – Cholera in Yemen

There were 1.2 million cases, and 2,500 people died.

2017-2023 – Lassa Fever in Nigeria

1103 people died.

2017 – Dengue in Pakistan

69 people died.

2017 – Japanese Encephalitis in India

1317 people died.

2017 – Dengue in Sri Lanka

440 people died.

2018 – Nipah Virus in India

17 people died.

2018 – The Kivu Ebola Epidemic

The epidemic began in the Democratic Republic of the Congo. By November 2018, the outbreak became the second-largest Ebola outbreak in recorded history. In 2019, the virus reached Uganda. The death toll was over 1,000.

2019 – Vaccine vs. Ebola

Ervebo is a recombinant, replication-competent vaccine using genetically engineered vesicular stomatitis virus to express a glycoprotein that provokes an immune response to Ebola.

2019 – Measles in The Congo

In 2019, measles infected 250,000 people in the Democratic Republic of the Congo and killed 5,000; most were children under five.

2019 – Measles in New Zealand

Thanks to prompt public health measures, only 2 people died.

2019 – Measles in the Philippines

415 people died.

2019 – Measles in Malaysia

15 people died.

2019 – Measles in Samoa

83 people died.

2019 – Dengue in Asia Pacific and Latin America

3931 people died.

2019 – Polio Eradication Stalls

Clusters erupted in Afghanistan and Pakistan after anti-vaccine protesters killed a vaccinator. Additionally, polio reemerged in Iran, Nigeria, Somalia, Ghana, Benin, Chad, Niger, Togo, the Democratic Republic of the Congo, Angola, the Central African Republic, China, the Philippines, Zambia, Malaysia, and Myanmar.

2019-2022 - The COVID-19 Pandemic

In 2015, Vineet D Menachery, Boyd L Yount Jr, et al. published an article in *Nature Medicine* (VOLUME 21, NUMBER 12, DECEMBER 2015). It warned that coronaviruses can replicate in humans and that there was a potential risk of a SARS or MERS epidemic in the future. Yet, despite the warning, no country began preparations for the possibility of an epidemic.

In September 2019, 959 Italian patients had blood samples taken and stored for future research. When Giovanni Apolone, Emanuele Montomoli, and Alessandro Manenti examined the samples in March 2021, they found SARS-CoV-2 (COVID-19) antibodies in 111 samples.

Unexpected detection of SARS-CoV-2 antibodies in pre-pandemic Italy
https://journals.sagepub.com/doi/full/10.1177/0300891620974755

Tumori. 2021 Mar 22:300891620987756.
https://doi.org/10.1177/03008916209747 55

Author's note: the article above was first published in Tumori on November 11, 2020. It was then subject to an expression of concern on March 22, 2021. The expression of concern was removed in June 2021.

Thus, *in retrospect*, SARS-CoV-2 <u>may</u> have already been in Italy three months *before* the world's first case was identified.

The world first learned about COVID-19 on December 8, 2019. That day, in Wuhan, China, a woman contracted an unusual pneumonia and spread it to others. On December 26, 2019, Jixian Zhang, MD, director of the Respiratory and Critical Care Department at Hubei Provincial Hospital, treated four cases of the new pneumonia, all within the same family. She reported the situation to the local CDC. Three more patients appeared on December 30, 2019, and China's CDC notified WHO on December 31, 2019. By January 7, 2020, scientists in China had mapped the RNA of the mutated coronavirus, known as SARS-CoV-2.

Despite unprecedented quarantine measures in China and other countries, the disease quickly spread worldwide. A traveler from Wuhan was the first U.S. case in January 2020.

By March, 163 countries reported 250,000 cases with 10,000 deaths. In April, there were one million cases in 183 countries, with 55,000 deaths. By May, it had infected 5.8 million people and caused 363,000 deaths. The USA had 1.7 million cases and 102,000 deaths. In September 2020, nine months after it started, the epidemic infected thirty-three million worldwide, with one million deaths. The U.S. reported seven million infected and 200,000 deaths.

By November 2020, U.S. infections were twelve million, with 250,000 deaths. Worldwide, there were 58.7 million cases and 1.38 million deaths.

By January 2021, COVID-19 had infected one hundred million people worldwide, resulting in two million deaths. In the U.S., there were twenty-six million infections and 400,000 deaths.

The World Health Organization estimated a need for two billion doses of a COVID-19 vaccine. In the U.S., Operation Warp Speed funded $10 billion for 300 million vaccine doses. By December 2020, forty-four vaccines were being tested for initial safety and dosage, nineteen were in expanded safety trials, eighteen were undergoing large-scale efficacy tests, and five were in limited use. The U.S. approved two in December and began widespread vaccinations in January 2021.

By June 2021, eighteen months into the pandemic, 34 million documented cases in the USA had resulted in 600,000 deaths. Globally, at least 200 million cases caused 4 million deaths. A large effort vaccinated 40 percent (135 million) of the U.S. population, and daily deaths dropped to "only" 700. However, 94% of the world still remained unvaccinated.

The massive worldwide reservoir of COVID-19 infections generated innumerable mutations. For example, Delta emerged in India in December 2020 and rapidly spread throughout that country and Great Britain before reaching the U.S., where it quickly surged.

Delta soon accounted for more than 99% of COVID-19 cases, leading to an overwhelming increase in hospitalizations and ICU admissions. Additionally, Delta was significantly more contagious than the original strain, with an R0 factor of approximately eight.

By January 2021, COVID-19 had infected one hundred million globally, with two million deaths. America had twenty-three million infected and 380,000 dead.

As of July 11, 2022, COVID-19 has caused more than 6 million excess deaths.

Scientists rushed forty-four vaccines into testing, and widespread vaccinations began in early 2021.

No effective treatment or cure was available for the pandemic's first years. In 2021, the European Medicines Agency's Committee for Medicinal Products for Human Use approved Paxlovid (nirmatrelvir plus ritonavir) for the treatment of adults. In the US, the FDA later granted it Emergency Use Authorization.

Unfortunately, opportunists profited by spreading misinformation about the disease and vaccines through social media.

COVID-19 vaccines were widely distributed in various countries after December 2020. According to a June 2022 study, COVID-19 vaccines prevented 17 million deaths from 2020 to 2021.

As of November 2022, 27 million excess deaths had been caused by COVID-19.

The **COVID-19** pandemic caused widespread social and economic disruption, as well as the most significant global recession since the Great Depression. Additionally, widespread supply and food shortages occurred.

2020 – Nobel Prize for Medicine

The 2020 Nobel Prize in Physiology or Medicine went to Harvey J. Alter, Michael Houghton, and Charles M. Rice for discovering the Hepatitis C virus. They made blood tests for the virus possible and virtually ended post-transfusion hepatitis.

2020 – Ebola in the Congo

55 people died.

2020 – Dengue in Singapore

32 people died.

2020 – Yellow Fever hits Nigeria

296 people died.

2021 – Mucormycosis (Black Fungus) in India

4332 people died.

2022 – Monkeypox Worldwide

280 people died.

2022 – Ebola in Uganda

77 people died.

2023 – Legionella in Poland

23 people died.

2023 – Dengue in Brazil

1625 people died.

2023 – 2025 – World-Wide Mpox

812 people died.

2023 – 2025 – Sudanese Cholera Epidemic

5869 people died in Sudan, South Sudan, and Chad.

Bibliography

Abbasi, Jennifer. 2021. *The Flawed Science of Antibody Testing for SARS-CoV-2 Immunity.* JAMA. 2021;326(18):1781-1782.

Apolone, Montomoli, Manenti, Boeri, Sabia, Hyseni, Mazzini, Martinuzzi, Cantone, Milanese. *Unexpected Detection of SARS-CoV-2 Antibodies in the Pre-pandemic Period in Italy.*

Arnold, Catharine. 2018. *Pandemic 1918: Eyewitness Accounts from the Greatest Medical Holocaust in Modern History.* St. Martin's Publishing Group.

Barry, John M. 2004. *The Great Influenza: The Story of the Deadliest Pandemic in History.* Penguin Books.

Chakraborty, Tirtha. 2008. *Dengue Fever and Other Hemorrhagic Viruses.* Chelsea House Publications.

Coleman, William. 2009. *Cholera.* Chelsea House Publications.

Crosby, Alfred W. 1072. *The Columbian Exchange, Biological and Cultural Consequences of 1492.* Greenwood Publishing Group. ISBN978-0837172286

Defoe, Daniel. 1722. *History of the Plague in London.* https://www.gutenberg.org/ebooks/17221

Defoe, Daniel. 1723. *A Journal of the Plague Year, Written by a Citizen Who Continued All the While in London.* https://www.gutenberg.org/ebooks/376

Dorwart, Bonnie Brice. 2010. *Death Is in the Breeze: Disease During the American Civil War.* National Museum of Civil War Medicine.

Emmeluth, Donald, I. Edward Alcamo, and David L. Heymann. 2009. *Typhoid Fever*. Infobase Publishing.

Freeman, Henry. 2016. *The Black Death: History's Most Effective Killer*. CreateSpace Independent Publishing Platform.

Griffin, Diane E. 2008. *Measles: History and Basic Biology*. Springer.

Griffin, Diane E., and Michael B. A. Oldstone. 2008. *Measles: Pathogenesis and Control*. Springer.

Grob, Gerald N. 2002. *The Deadly Truth: A History of Disease in America*. 1st edition. Cambridge, MA: Harvard University Press.

Hempel, Sandra. 2018. *The Atlas of Disease: Mapping Deadly Epidemics and Contagion from the Plague to the Zika Virus*. White Lion Publishing.

Humphreys, Margaret. 1999. *Yellow Fever and the South*. Revised ed. edition. Baltimore, Md: JHUP.

Johnson, Steven. 2007. *The Ghost Map: The Story of London's Most Terrifying Epidemic - and How It Changed Science, Cities, and the Modern World*. Illustrated edition. London: Riverhead Books.

Johnson, Steven. 2007. *The Ghost Map: The Story of London's Most Terrifying Epidemic--and How It Changed Science, Cities, and the Modern World*. Illustrated edition. London: Riverhead Books.

Kang, Lydia, and Nate Pedersen. 2017. *Quackery: A Brief History of the Worst Ways to Cure Everything*. Workman Publishing.

Kelly, John. 2006. *The Great Mortality: An Intimate History of the Black Death, the Most Devastating Plague of All Time*. Reprint edition. New York, NY: Harper Perennial.

Kruel, Donald. 2007. *Trypanosomiasis*. Infobase Publishing.

Li, Carroll, Gardner, Walsh, Vitalis, Damon. *On the Origin of Smallpox: Correlating Variola Phylogenics with Historical Smallpox Records*.

McEleney, Brenda J. 2000. *Smallpox: A Primer*. USAF Counterproliferation Center, Air University.

McEleney, Brenda J. 2000. *Smallpox: A Primer*. USAF Counterproliferation Center, Air University.

McMillen, Christian W. 2016. *Pandemics: A Very Short Introduction*. Very Short Introduction, 1.0. Oxford University Press.

Oldstone, Michael B. A. 1998. *Viruses, Plagues, and History*. Oxford University Press.

Oshinsky, David M. 2006. *Polio: An American Story*. Illustrated edition. Oxford; New York: Oxford University Press.

Parker, Steve, Alexandra Black, Philip Parker, Sally Regan, and Marcus Weeks. 2016. *Medicine: The Definitive Illustrated History*. DK.

Porter, Roy. 1999. *The Greatest Benefit to Mankind: A Medical History of Humanity (The Norton History of Science)*. W. W. Norton & Company.

Powell, J. H., Kenneth R. Foster, Mary F. Jenkins, and Anna Coxe Toogood. 1993. *Bring Out Your Dead: The*

Great Plague of Yellow Fever in Philadelphia in 1793. Philadelphia: University of Pennsylvania Press.

Riedel, MD, Ph.D., Stefan. 2005. *Edward Jenner and the History of Smallpox and Vaccination.* Proc Baylor Univ Medical Center. 2005 Jan; 18(1): 21–25. https://www.ncbi.nlm.nih.gov/pmc/articles/PMC1200696/

River, Charles. 2020. *John Snow and the Cholera Epidemic of 1854: The History of the Outbreak and Its Impact on Public Health Measures.* Charles River Editors.

River, Charles. 2020. *The Roman Empire and the Plague: The History of the Worst Pandemics to Strike Rome and the Byzantines in Antiquity and the Middle Ages.* Independently Published.

River, Charles. 2020. *Fighting the Plague in Antiquity and the Middle Ages: The History of Ancient and Medieval Efforts to Prevent the Spread of Diseases.* Charles River Editors.

River, Charles. 2020. *John Snow and the Cholera Epidemic of 1854: The History of the Outbreak and Its Impact on Public Health Measures.* Charles River Editors.

Roossinck, Marilyn J. 2016. *Virus: An Illustrated Guide to 101 Incredible Microbes.* Princeton University Press.

Rosenberg, Charles E. 1987. *The Cholera Years: The United States in 1832, 1849, and 1866.* 2nd edition. Chicago: University of Chicago Press.

Sandra Hempel. 2018. *The Atlas of Disease: Mapping Deadly Epidemics and Contagion from the Plague to the Zika Virus.* White Lion Publishing.

Saracci, Rodolfo. 2010. *Epidemiology: A Very Short Introduction*. Very Short Introduction, 1.0. OUP Oxford.

Schneider, David. 2021. *The Invention of Surgery: A History of Modern Medicine: From the Renaissance to the Implant Revolution*. Pegasus Books.

Shmaefsky, Brian R. 2009. *Yellow Fever*. Infobase Publishing.

Slack, Paul. 2012. *Plague: A Very Short Introduction*. Oxford University Press.

Willrich, Michael. 2011. *Pox: An American History*. The Penguin Press.

Willrich, Michael. 2011. *Pox: An American History*. The Penguin Press.

Yount, Boyd L, Kari Debbink, Sudhakar Agnihothram, Lisa E Gralinski, Jessica A Plante, Rachel L Graham, Trevor Scobey, et al. 2019. *A SARS-like Cluster of Circulating Bat Coronaviruses Shows Potential for Human Emergence*. Nature Publishing Group.

Books by James R. Jones

Anger
A Contented Life, Practical Advice from Stoicism
Surviving in Management
Healthcare Contracting for Physician Executives
A Brief Outline of the History of Medicine
5000 Years of Plagues
Our Recipes
Camp Canoe Kayak – 50 Years of Wilderness Water Trips

amazon.com/author/jamesrjones

www.ingramcontent.com/pod-product-compliance
Lightning Source LLC
Chambersburg PA
CBHW070349220526
45467CB00001B/304